Background and Management of Muscular Atrophy

Edited by Julianna Cseri

Published in London, United Kingdom

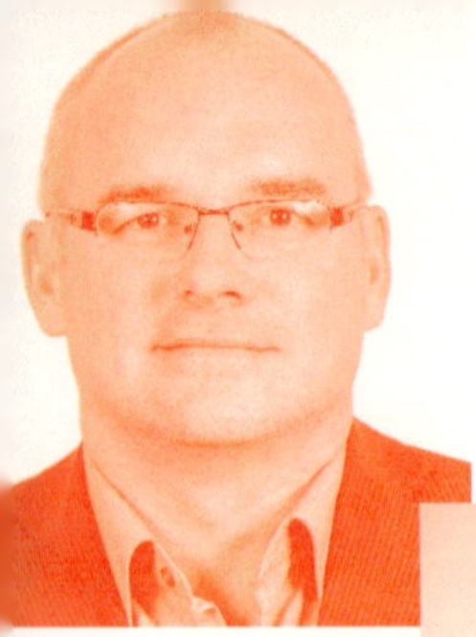
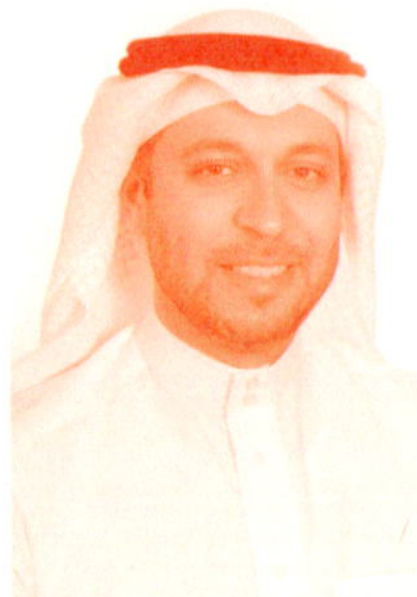
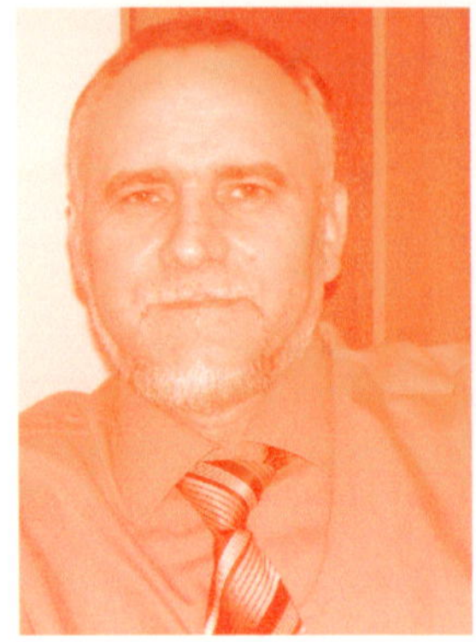
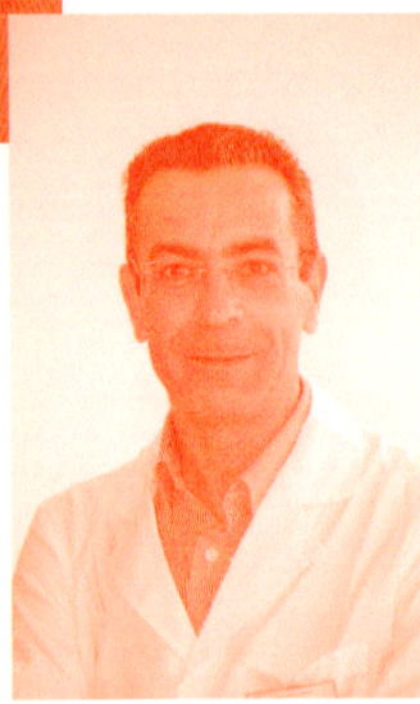
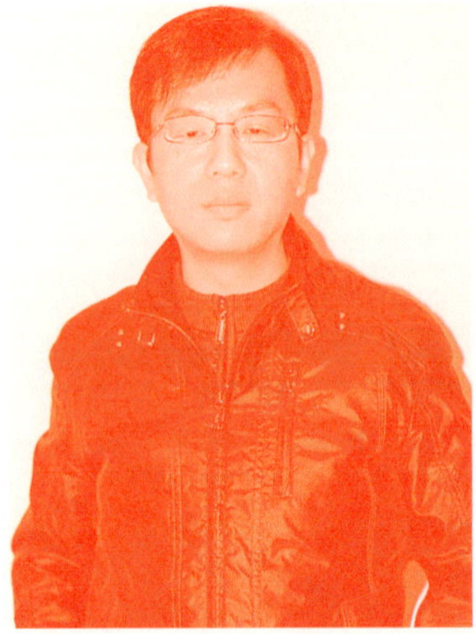
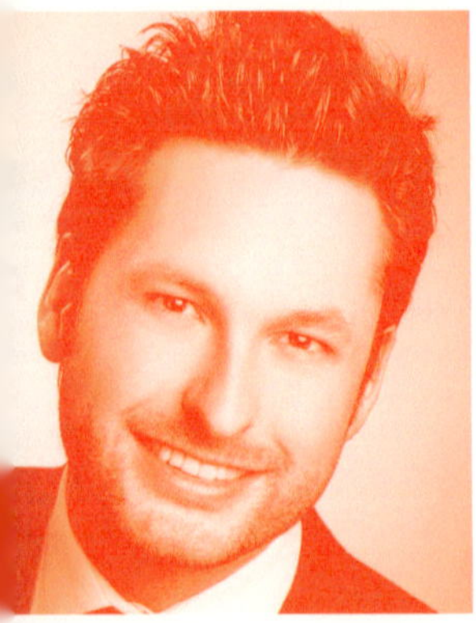
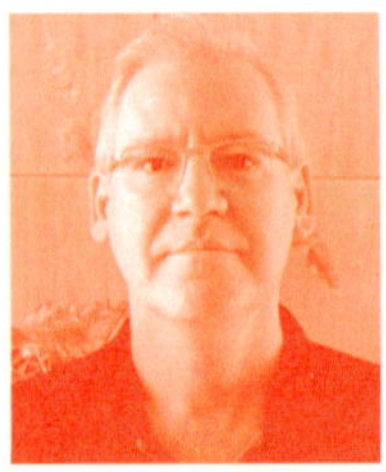

IntechOpen

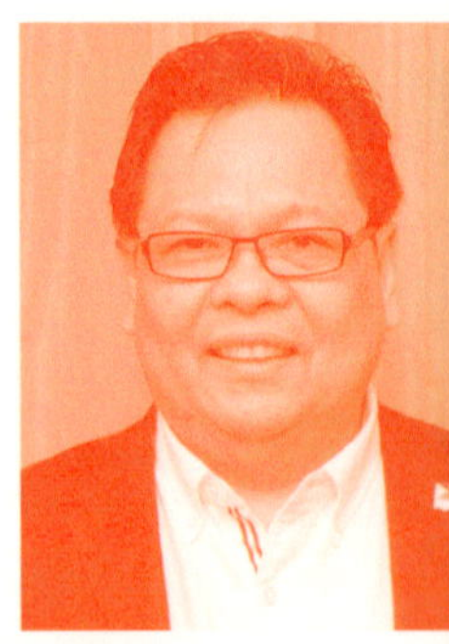
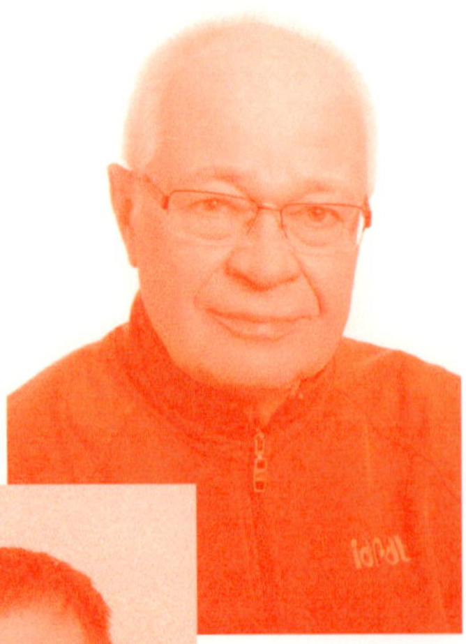
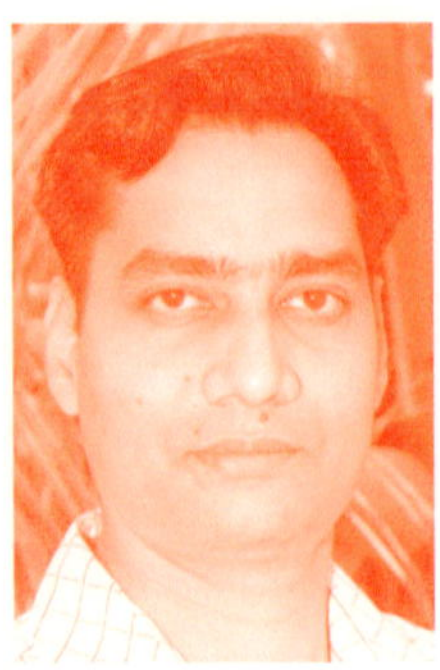
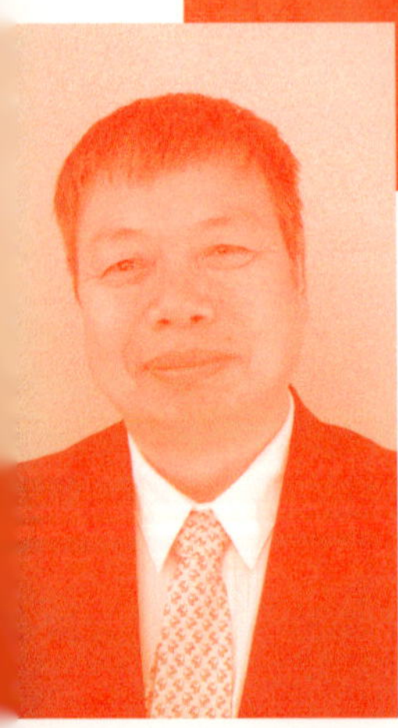
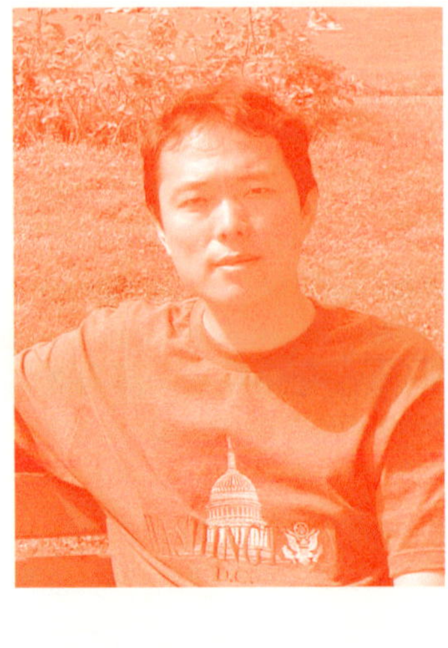
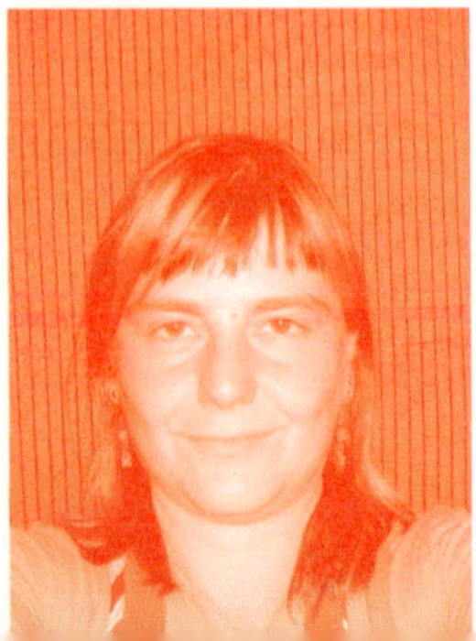

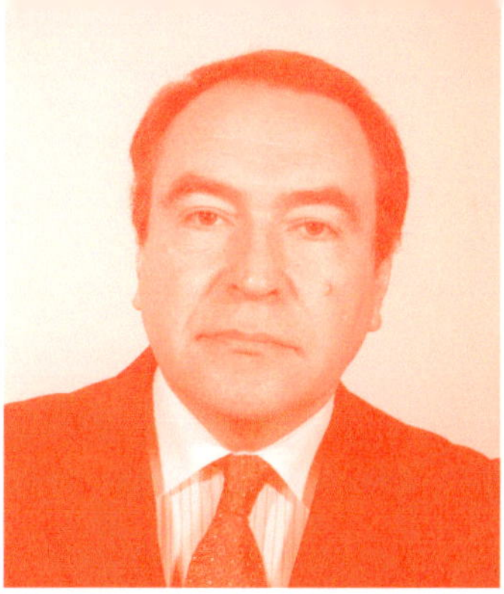
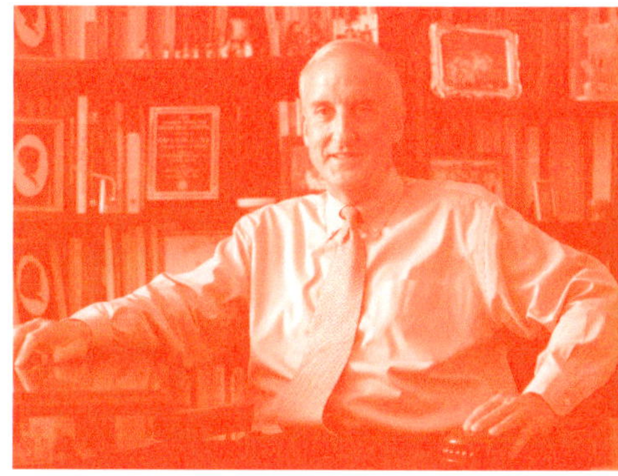
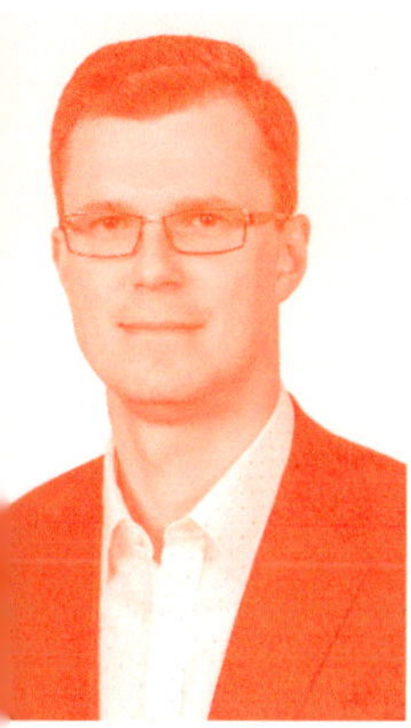
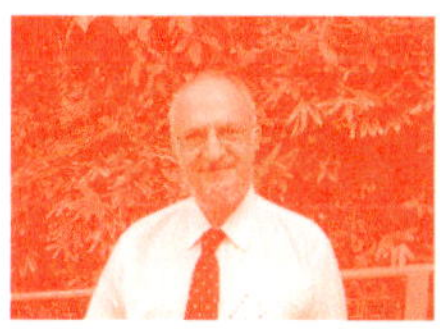
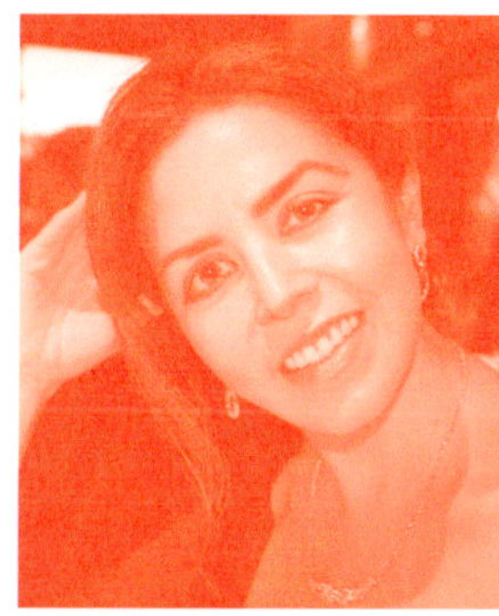

Supporting open minds since 2005

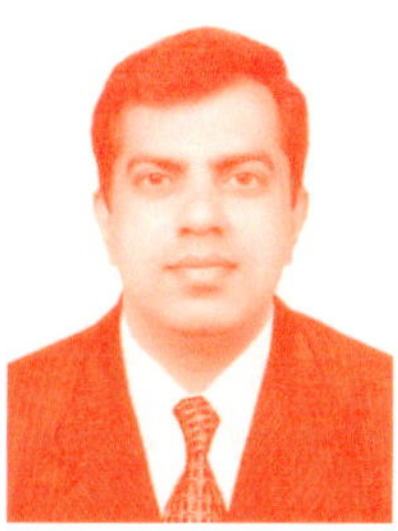
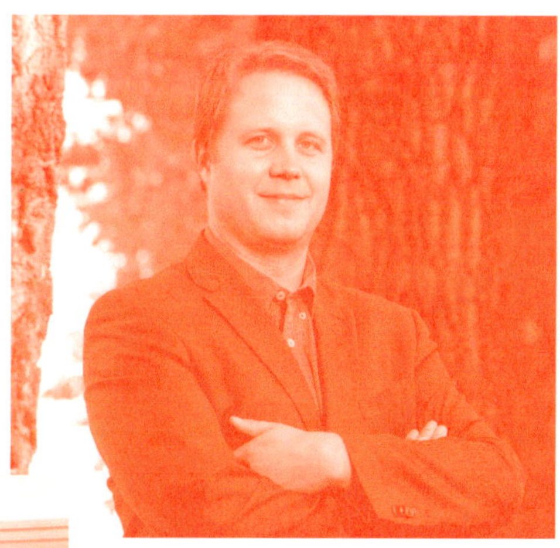
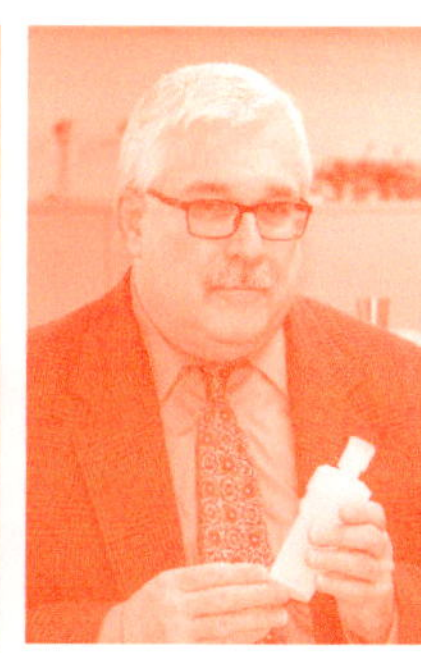
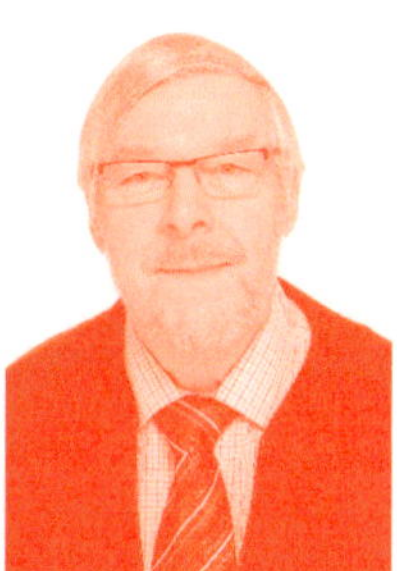
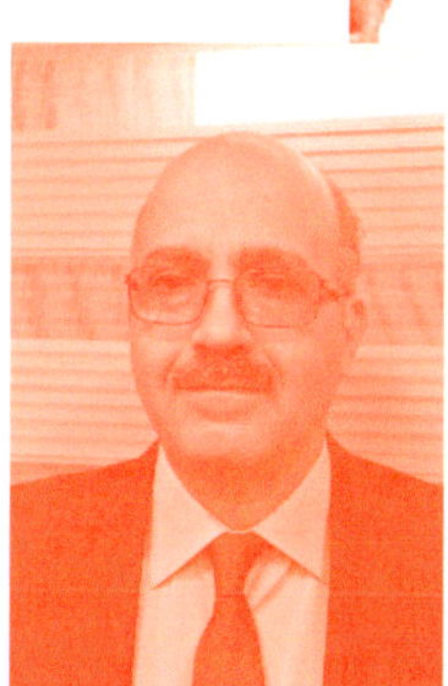
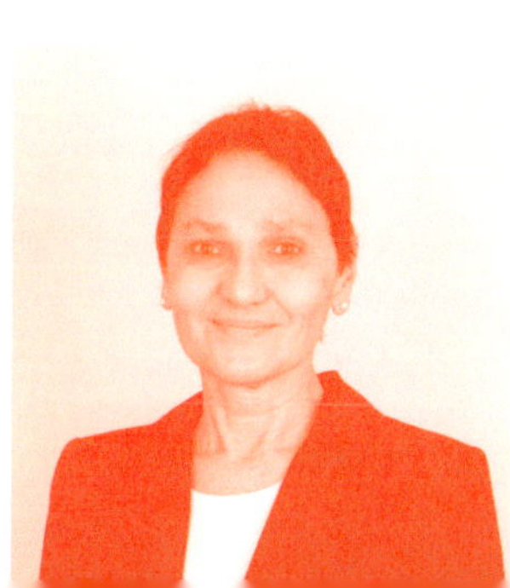
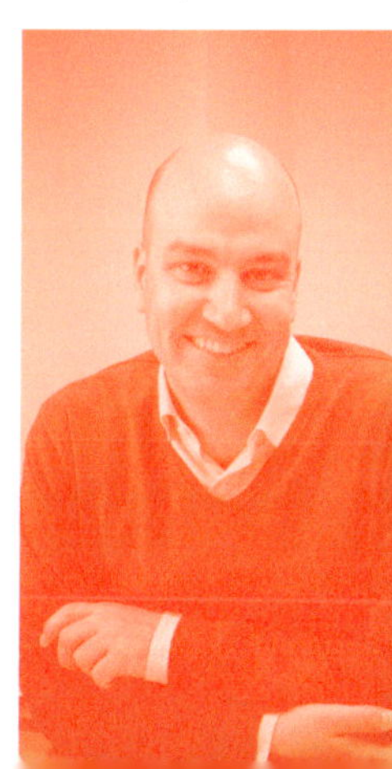

Background and Management of Muscular Atrophy
http://dx.doi.org/10.5772/intechopen.90959
Edited by Julianna Cseri

Contributors
Eli Carmeli, Suka Aryana, Mohit Kwatra, Sahabuddin Ahmed, Vgm Naidu, Samir Ranjan Panda, Nitika Gupta, Muneshige Shimizu, Kunihiro Sakuma, Tsan-Hon Liou, Chun-De Liao, Shih-Wei Huang, Guo Cheng, Quanjun Yang, Chen Linlin, Hong Zhang, Mengyi Chi, Viany Anggi, Boglárka Debity, Julianna Cseri, Sanda M. Cretoiu, Madalina-Garbriela Barbu, Andreea-Elena Boboc, Lidia Filip, Oana-Larisa Bugnar, Dragos Cretoiu, Nicolae Suciu, Silviu-Cristian Voinea, Daniela Oana Toader

First published in London, United Kingdom, 2021 by IntechOpen
IntechOpen is the global imprint of INTECHOPEN LIMITED, registered in England and Wales, registration number: 11086078, 5 Princes Gate Court, London, SW7 2QJ, United Kingdom
Printed in Croatia

British Library Cataloguing-in-Publication Data
A catalogue record for this book is available from the British Library

Additional hard and PDF copies can be obtained from orders@intechopen.com

Background and Management of Muscular Atrophy
Edited by Julianna Cseri
p. cm.
Print ISBN 978-1-83880-724-5
Online ISBN 978-1-83880-725-2
eBook (PDF) ISBN 978-1-83880-726-9

For EU product safety concerns:
IN TECH d.o.o., Prolaz Marije Krucifikse Kozulić 3, 51000 Rijeka, Croatia, info@intechopen.com or visit our website at intechopen.com.

Meet the editor

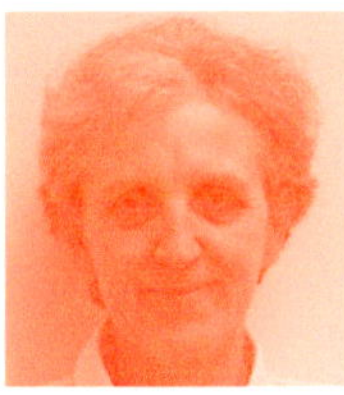

Julianna Cseri, M.D., Ph.D., is a College Professor retired from the Department of Physiotherapy, Faculty of Public Health, University of Debrecen, Debrecen, Hungary. Her scientific field is skeletal muscle physiology. She was awarded her general medicine diploma in 1973 from the University Medical School of Debrecen and started scientific work at the Department of Physiology, University Medical School of Debrecen (later the Faculty of Medicine University of Debrecen). She achieved scientific qualifications in muscle electrophysiology. Her attention was later turned to the proliferation and differentiation of the skeletal muscle in cell cultures and the role of intracellular calcium homeostasis in myogenesis. This work is closely related to muscle degeneration and regeneration in vivo, managed by physiotherapy interventions.

Contents

Preface

The loss of skeletal muscle mass and strength substantially impairs physical performance and the quality of life, especially in older patients. The prevention and treatment of muscle atrophy is a big challenge for clinicians and other professionals. The book chapters provide insight into the molecular, morphological, and functional changes under conditions that lead to muscular atrophy. The sarcopenia in older patients is highlighted in many chapters. The normal situation and the age-related changes in the motor unit (motor neuron, neuromuscular junction, and skeletal muscle) are demonstrated and the role of impaired bone remodeling are presented in some chapters. Other chapters present and discuss the tools for the management of muscular atrophy (sarcopenia) in older patients and other types of muscular atrophy. The pharmacological, nutritional, and physiotherapeutic approaches are demonstrated in detail, as well as the possible role of herbal antioxidants in the treatment of muscular atrophy. The chapters may be interesting for professionals in clinical practice, for medical and health care students as well as for researchers working in muscle-related fields of science.

Special thanks to Romina Rovan, Author Service Manager, for professional guidance during the whole editing process.

Julianna, Cseri
Department of Physiotherapy,
University of Debrecen,
Debrecen, Hungary

Section 1

Molecular Mechanisms of Muscular Atrophy and Age-related Changes in Skeletal Muscle Structure and Function

Chapter 1

Molecular Mechanisms, Therapeutic Targets and Pharmacological Interventions: An Update

Mohit Kwatra, Sahabuddin Ahmed, Samir Ranjan Panda, Vegi Ganga Modi Naidu and Nitika Gupta

Abstract

Muscles are the enriched reservoir of proteins in the body. During any workout or exercise, the demand in the form of energy is essentially required by the muscle. Energy expenditure of skeletal muscle is more dependent on the type of demand. There is particular homeostasis within the body that avoid surplus energy expenditure and this prevents any muscle loss. Muscle atrophy is termed as the loss of skeletal muscle mass due to immobility, malnutrition, medications, aging, cancer cachexia, variety of injuries or diseases that impact the musculoskeletal or nervous system. Hence, atrophy within the skeletal muscle initiates further cause fatigue, pain, muscle weakness, and disability in human subjects. Therefore, starvation and reduced muscle mass further initiate numerous signaling pathways including inflammatory, antioxidant signaling, mitochondria bio-energetic failure, AMP-activated protein kinase (AMPK), Sirtuin 1(SIRT1), BDNF/TrkB/PKC, Autophagy, ubiquitin-proteasome systems, etc. Here, in this chapter, we will mention molecular mechanisms involved in therapeutic targets and available Pharmacological Interventions with the latest updates.

Keywords: molecular mechanisms, therapeutic targets, pharmacological Interventions

1. Introduction

Muscles are enormous protein reservoirs within the body. It is a profound source of various amino acids required for energy production used by various organs (such as brain, liver, heart) during energy demand and disease conditions (cancer, AIDS, burn, heart failure). However, extensive protein requirement does not consider good in case of cachexia which might lead to increased morbidity and mortality. Skeletal muscle is an organ with plastic characteristics and regulated by several signaling pathways that control cell and protein turnover. The skeletal muscle atrophy may be due to lower muscle mass, disease. However, disuse muscle mediated acute atrophy is reversed through exercise. Furthermore, chronic atrophy such as sarcopenia features as loss of muscle mass strength with age. Moreover, other chronic diseases such as diabetes or disease of muscles (muscle dystrophy) cause nerve damage to innervate to the muscle [1]. In muscle atrophy, a proteolytic system gets activated while contractile proteins and organelles are removed results in the shrinkage of muscle fibers.

Spinal muscular atrophy (SMA), a kind of intense neuromuscular disease depicts as chief genetic cause of death in infants. It is featured as alpha motor neuron degeneration within the anterior horn region of the spinal cord and brain stem that is the leading cause of progressive muscle weakness. SMA is inherited as autosomal recessive disorder and the most common form (95% cases) caused by certain mutations in the survival motor neuron 1 (*SMN1, SMN*^{T}) gene localized on chromosome 5q12.2. The genetic deletion or carries a mutation of the SMN1 gene resulting SMN protein deficit. On the other hand, the SMN2 gene develops a relatively small amount of functional SMN protein and SMN2 copy numbers further determine the severity of the disease. The incidence of SMA is approx. 1 in 10,000 live births while prevalence estimates 1–2 in 100,000 affected individuals with extremely shortened life expectancy. SMA characterizes in various forms depending on the age of inception such as Infants being severely hypotonic possess feeding problems, further reach growing age of children does found with difficulty climbing stairs proceeded with frequent falls. The clinical manifestation of SMA is usually heterogeneous and scored to a range from severe to mild phenotype which is further divided into mainly 3 subtypes as Type I (also known as Werdnig-Hoffmann disease), type II and, type III (also called Kugelberg Welander disease). SMA categorized as type 0, a serious and rigorous form, lower/absent movements, abnormal muscle contractions, and immediate need for ventilation support. SMA type IV, a mild late (adult) onset [2]. Hence, improve understanding regarding the molecular pathogenesis mechanisms cause for muscle atrophy or muscle wasting attribute the efforts to designate the safe and effective therapy for affected human subjects.

2. Molecular key mechanisms in muscle and spinal muscular atrophy

Various signaling pathways participate in molecular pathogenesis of muscle atrophy **(Figure 1)**.

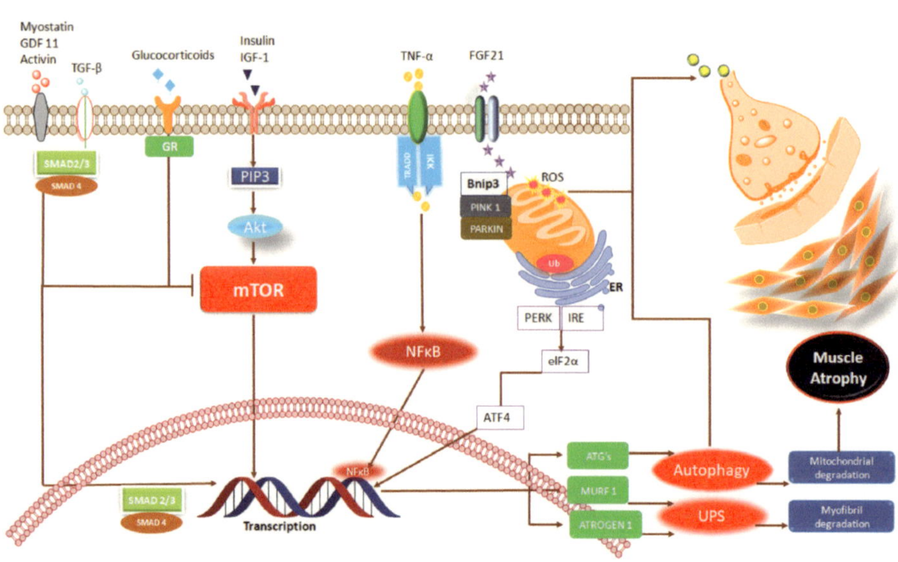

Figure 1.
Signaling Cascade Events in Muscle Atrophy.

2.1 Oxidative stress and inflammatory signaling

Oxidative stress and inflammation are considered the foremost molecular mechanisms responsible for muscle atrophy [3]. Raised levels of reactive oxygen species (ROS) production within skeletal muscles substantially promote mitochondrial function impairment, stimulate forkhead box class O (FoxO) transcription factors leads to inactivity induced muscle atrophy [4]. Inflammation perturbs the muscle homeostasis and process of myogenesis via activating the family of FoxO transcription factors significantly contribute to skeletal muscle atrophy [5]. FoxO activation is vital for the muscle atrophy induced through denervation/fasting, which upon activation (FoxO3) cause induction of ubiquitin–proteasome system (UPS) and autophagy–lysosomal system (ALS) in a coordinate manner, especially lysosomal proteolysis [6]. Shreds of evidence, state that FoxO knockout was able to reverse the muscle degeneration process loss, also the markers of increased UPS process and autophagy dysfunction in streptozotocin-diabetes induced mice (O'Neill et al., 2019). Therefore, necessary steps must be taken to find an intervention that can curb the atrophy. During muscle wasting or cachexia, NFκB transcription factors activate with certain stimulants or facilitators (such as TNF-α). Upon TNFα response, the IκB complex gets phosphorylates by IκB kinase (IKKβ), ensuing ubiquitylation followed by its proteasomal degradation which further causes nuclear translocation of NFκB and induce transcription of inflammatory mediators [7]. Transgenic mice showing muscle-specific overexpression of IKKβ results in drastic muscle wasting due to ubiquitin ligase MuRF1 and not by atrogin-1 [8]. Furthermore, muscle-specific inhibition of NFκB through transgenic expression of a typically active IκB mutant generated partial results due to denervation atrophy get substantially reduced [9]. Besides, mice deficient with p105/p50 subunit of NFκB reduced hindlimb unloading induced muscle atrophy [4, 10]. The pro-inflammatory cytokines including TNF-α cause insulin resistance and repress the Insulin-like growth factor-AKT (IGF1-Akt) pathway [11]. Furthermore, hyperphosphorylation of AKT was found in IKKβ knockout mouse which develops resistance against muscular atrophy [12]. These findings signify the important crosstalk of two pathways, and further future studies are desirable for elucidating respective links of the IKKβ-NFκB and Akt-FoxO pathways in muscle atrophy.

Moreover, an inflammatory cytokine strongly concerned for muscle-wasting disease is the TNF-like weak inducer of apoptosis (TWEAK), which binds on the surface receptor FN14 and induces NF-κB activation. TWEAK deficient mice ablate atrophy upon denervation, a process that generally activates TWEAK [13, 14]. Furthermore, the TWEAK-F14 axis may be a potential therapeutic target in muscle wasting diseases [15].

2.2 Mitochondrial dysfunction

Mitochondrial functional impairment is a critical regulatory event that brings on activation of atrophic programs in inactivity-induced muscle atrophy. Prolonged muscle inactivity induces mitochondria suffers from prompt reduction in the respiratory capacity, coupling, lower mitochondrial volume, mitochondrial ROS overload, and destruct mitochondrial architectures. Muscle inactivity, promotes mitochondrial fission rather than fusion and therefore decays energy level and leads to muscle atrophy [16, 17].

Mitochondrial fusion and fission process need excessive refinement due to mitochondrial lipid bilayer hence need synchronization at inner as well as outer membrane. Upon fusion process, mitofusin1 and 2 (MFN1 and MFN2) proteins facilitate fusion by attaching to an outer membrane in adjoining mitochondria, while the inner membranes by optic atrophy 1 (OPA1). Additionally, MFN 1 and 2 also functions over junctions to create membrane-associated-sarcoplasmic reticulum membranes (MAM) to play keen role in mitochondrial Ca^{2+} management. Further, a major regulative component that regulate fusion with MFN proteins is the E3 ligase Parkin, which ubiquitinates MFN1 and MFN2 cause its extraction from the outer membrane of mitochondria with subsequent degradation and thereby prevent mitochondrial fusion [18, 19]. The mitochondrial fission is largely coordinated by dynamin-related protein 1 (DRP1). DRP1 locates in the cytosol and upon certain signaling event, process induce it translocate to the outer mitochondrial membrane. Phosphorylation at Ser616 is believed to activate DRP1, while phosphorylation at Ser637 and Ser693 inactivate DRP1 and prevention of mitochondrial fission activity altered through sumoylation and S-nitrosylation [20]. The muscle inactivity results in alterations of the proteins involve in both fusion and fission [21]. Inactivity-mediated muscle atrophy leads to increased total as well as phosphorylated (i.e., pDRP1-S616, active) DRP1 which explains it as an essential mediator of the mitochondrial division. Additionally, MFN1, MFN2, and OPA1 function as fusion promoters is found lower in protein content and hence limit the mitochondrial fusion process while promote mitochondrial fission.

Peroxisome proliferator-activated receptor gamma coactivator 1-alpha (PGC-1α), a key regulator of mitochondrial biogenesis is found significantly decreased with prolonged muscle immobility. PGC-1α, a transcriptional coactivator assists the regulation of genes involved in mitochondrial biogenesis, fatty acid oxidation, and glycolysis. The reduction in PGC-1α abundance markedly impaired mitochondrial biogenesis negatively influences mitochondrial structure and function. However, PGC-1α overexpression preserved mitochondria and improved muscle performance [22]. Furthermore, overexpression of PGC-1α ameliorates decreased MFN1, MFN2, and OPA1 in muscle wasting. This further outlooked the importance of upstream transcriptional activators [23, 24]. Importantly, muscle inactivity-induced dysfunctions in skeletal muscle mitochondria through elevations in mitochondrial ROS emission, the release of proteolytic-activating mitochondrial proteins, and triggering apoptotic cellular signaling cascade caused due to mitochondrial fragmentation [24].

2.3 TrκB/BDNF/PKC pathway

Neurotrophins always have been thought to work within neuronal cells and function as differentiators, nerve growth, neuronal survival, and apoptosis regulators [25–27]. Various evidence state that these neurotrophins have a diverse function in numerous cell populations across multiple tissue compartments than earlier thought. Among these, skeletal muscle seeks great importance as it act as a plentiful source with neurotrophic support throughout the development process. Neurotrophin knockout mice show unique defects in muscle growth and function. For instance, NT (4/5), NT-3 implicates for muscle fiber transformation and spindle formation and nerve growth factor (NGF) in muscle dystrophy [25]. Brain-derived neurotrophic factor (BDNF), a well-known member of the neurotrophin family, plays an utmost vital role in differentiation, synaptic plasticity, development, neuronal survival via activating tropomyosin-related kinase receptor B (TrkB) receptor. BDNF potentiates TrkB autophosphorylation leading to initiation of some signaling pathways, including the PI3K/Akt, Ras/Raf/ERK, and PLCγ/PKC.

Initially, BDNF is produced as a precursor (pro-BDNF), further cleaves to mBDNF (a mature isoform) by Intra/extracellular proteases. These two isoforms stimulate different and even opposite functions via interacting especially to low-affinity nerve growth factor receptor (p75) or the tropomyosin-related kinase B receptor (TrkB). Furthermore, alternative splicing of TrkB mRNA gives rise to a full-length TrkB isoform (TrkB.FL) and truncated TrkB isoforms T1 and T2 (TrkB.T1 and TrkB.T2) [28, 29]. TrkB.T1 is considered to be main truncated isoform in skeletal muscle tissue while TrkB.T2 (variant) chief variant function within brain regions. Growing evidence mentions that exercise training ensures CNS health, such as improving synaptic function. BDNF is secreted in an activity-dependent and its expression in the rodent spinal cord and skeletal muscle surges after a physical workout. Correspondingly, normal levels of neuromuscular activity are required to maintain basal levels of BDNF within the neuromuscular structure. Lastly, one study found that contracting cultured myotubes stimulated to release the BDNF and justify the postsynaptic origin (Matthews et al., 2009). However, the skeletal muscles release BDNF in *in-vivo* models, after contraction, either synaptic activity provokes its liberation, or a combination of both, the exact mechanisms remains elusive. Exogenous BDNF intensifies acetylcholine (ACh) discharge at neuromuscular junction via coupling with TrkB receptor This supports well where neuromuscular activity endorses BDNF/TrkB retrograde signaling in maintaining neuromuscular function [28, 30]. Furthermore, the nerve-stimulated muscle contraction is a chief regulator of the BDNF/TrkB signaling pathway, retrogradely activate conventional protein kinase C (cPKC) isoforms (in particular cPKCβI) in modifying synaptic function [31].

With embryonic development, primordial skeletal muscle cells express comparative higher BDNF levels and later downregulates with maturation. Furthermore, expression of BDNF does associate with myofibers development, which later expresses myosin heavy chain IIB. BDNF was also found regulating food intake and blood glucose level in genetically modified (*db/db*) obese mice [32]. Thus, it is obvious that BDNF drivesregulatory role in neurobiology and metabolism. Recent reports established the fact that physical activity (exercise) raises the circulating BDNF levels in healthy humans as well as patients of multiple sclerosis, nevertheless cellular sources still vague. Certain reports evidenced the increased BDNF mRNA transcriptome within skeletal muscle in response to muscle contraction, however, this substantiates the fact with BDNF source within neurons does innervate skeletal muscle compartments. A Contrasting study explains the BDNF mRNA expresses in skeletal muscle of murine and was found increased with inhibiting histone deacetylases (HDACs) [33]. Physical exercise also tends to block histone deacetylases and contracted muscles release BDNF and mentions as novel contraction-induced myokine [34]. Moreover, BDNF was found to possess metabolic activity in the skeletal muscle. It increased phosphorylation of AMPK, acetyl-coenzyme A carboxylase β (ACCβ), and raised the level of fatty acid oxidation studied *in vitro*, *in-vivo* (sex-dependent), and *ex vivo*. The impact of BDNF over fatty acid oxidation was AMPK-dependent, however, this increased energy regulation was found to repress inC2C12 cells infected with either AMPK dominant-negative form of adenovirus or employed AMPK inhibitor (Compound C). BDNF injected via electroporation within the tibialis cranialis muscle raises BDNF production and tropomyosin-related kinase B (TrkB$Tyr^{706/707}$) and extracellular signal-regulated protein kinase (p44/42 Thr^{202}/Tyr^{204}) phosphorylation. Also, phosphorylation of ACCβ was also noticed in BDNF electroporated muscles [35, 36]. This raises the possibility that BDNF analogs or BDNF mimetic drugs can be a possible therapeutic intervention in metabolic diseases.

In the case of spinal bulbar muscular atrophy (SBMA) which is an androgen-dependent neuromuscular disorder associates with polyglutamine expansion mutation in androgen receptor gene [37]. SMBA affects people with middle young age and is featured through persistent muscle weakness with lower androgen sensibility. The muscle-derived neurotrophic factors such as vascular endothelial growth factor (VEGF), neurotrophin-4, insulin-like growth factor-1 etc. expression is usually reduced in pathological condition and experimentally strengthen its expression within muscle improvised the condition in SBMA affected mice [37]. Further, a possible mechanism by which muscle-derived neurotrophic factors combat disease is by ameliorating it in retrograde axonal transport. The motor impairment in SBMA may disapprovingly depend upon lower levels of muscle-derived BDNF, concludes that neuromuscular function can be salvaged in disease condition via reloading with muscle BDNF. Probable locations of BDNF action for endorsing neuromuscular function are Schwann cells, motoneurons, and muscles. Despite muscle fiber or motor neurons gets damage, BDNF tends to promote regaining the function of residual motoneurons and muscle fibers as well. Nonetheless, the satellite cell population mobilize within muscle tissue is also induced by BDNF action [37].

2.4 SIRT1/AMPK/PGC-1α signaling

Starvation or energy deprivation limits glucose availability compensated by accelerating mitochondrial fatty acid oxidation within the skeletal muscle or peripheral tissues to reserve blood glucose amount and stream to the brain and red blood cells. Further, shortage of metabolic flexibility appropriately acclimatizes as per energy demands and nutrient availability forms a burden on energy homeostasis, resulting in the development of the metabolic disease. Such, metabolic transformations within the muscle are pushed towards synchronized transcriptional responses promote mitochondrial utilization of lipids as their substrates for the energy source. The variations in gene expression patterns are attained via the modulation of some transcriptional regulators such as coactivator PGC-1α and FOXO family of transcription factors, both are closely associated with the regulation of mitochondria and fatty acid metabolism [38, 39]. The activities of PGC-1α and FOXOs are seriously influenced by controlling their acetylation levels through the silent information regulator/Sirtuin (SIRT1) type III (NAD^+-dependent deacetylase). SIRT1 knock-down averts induction of mitochondrial/fat oxidation genes in glucose-limited myocytes.

AMP-activated protein kinase (AMPK), metabolic sensing protein is found robustly influence the transcriptional responses. It is a heterotrimeric Ser/Thr kinase consists of one catalytic (α) with another non-catalytic subunits (β and γ). Further, two different isoforms are the α and β subunits (α1 and α2 or β1 and β2), and the γ subunits are determined by different genes (γ1, γ2, and γ3). The γ subunits usually interact with AMP/ATP competitively and work jointly. The AMP binding surges the catalytic activity of complex and augments phosphorylation of Thr^{172}, crucial for activity. AMPK enhances SIRT1 activity by raising intracellular NAD+ levels. This leads to deacetylation of SIRT1 targets (NF-κB, PGC-1α, FOXO1) which corresponds physiological or pharmacological AMPK activation [40, 41]. Enhanced organ fibrosis comprises organ to malfunction in a variety of diseases. Tissue fibrosis is also an eminent pathological feature of dystrophic skeletal muscle seen in Duchenne muscular dystrophy (DMD) human subjects. Further, repression of muscle fibrosis may be a beneficial treatment strategy in patients suffers from muscular atrophy and dystrophy. Treatment with active flavonoid resveratrol suppresses interstitial fibrosis in the biceps femoris of *mdx* mice.

The muscle cells find to activate SIRT1 that reduces oxidative stress by preventing transforming growth factor-*β*- (TGF-*β*-) induced upregulation of NADPH oxidase (NOX), which congruently generates reactive oxygen species (ROS) [42]. SIRT1 inhibits inflammatory cascade mediator's transcription factors via carrying deacetylation of acetyl NF-κB to P-NFκB and repress inflammation within muscles. Furthermore, deacetylation of peroxisome proliferator-activated receptor gamma coactivator 1-alpha (PGC-1α) via SIRT1 induces transcription of mitochondrial and HIF2αgenes and hence promotes fast to slow fiber shift [43–45]. Tissue fibrosis is reduced by SIRT1 which function by two mechanisms in fibroblasts. One is SIRT1-mediated deacetylation and inhibition of Smad transcription factors. Secondly, p300 deacetylation by SIRT1 following p300 protein degradation by the ubiquitin-proteasome pathway. Hence, the anti-fibrotic effect linked to SIRT1 activation may be valuable in treating muscular dystrophies [44].

Silent information regulator 1 or sirtuin 1 (SIRT-1) have seemed as the auspicious target of these pathways. It was found inhibiting differentiation of mouse C2C12 myoblasts and then reduce myogenin expression, a chief regulator with myogenic speciality and differentiate activate satellite cells. Furthermore, SIRT-1 directly involves in proliferating satellite cells. The outcomes propose that SIRT-1 impart significant role to sustain or raise satellite cells proliferation [44]. Overexpression of SIRT-1 activates the PI3K/AKT/mTOR pathway or increases levels of JunB or PGC-1α and able to induce rapid growth. SIRT-1 excites growth within muscles by inhibiting basal protein degradation with minimal or no change in overall protein synthesis [46]. Though FoxOs induction is critical for proteolysis enhancement either by autophagy or ubiquitin-proteasome system (UPS) through muscle atrophy and hence, FoxO3 inhibition was observed with hypertrophy induction by increasing protein synthesis. SIRT1 activation inhibits atrophy while promote rapid muscle growth through inhibition of FoxOs and parallel activating PGC-1α, with appropriate therapeutic implication in muscle wasting diseases [46].

2.5 Ubiquitin-proteasome systems

Within muscles, the ubiquitin-proteasome system (UPS) functions as removing sarcomeric proteins with changing muscle performance [4]. Lower muscle mass is related to (1) raised attachment of ubiquitin to muscle proteins; (2) overactive proteasome ATP dependent activity; (3) higher proteolysis (4) increased transcripts encoding ubiquitin, some ubiquitin-conjugating enzymes (E2), a few ubiquitin-protein ligases (E3) along with several proteasome subunits. E1 enzymes induce ubiquitin proteins after cleaving ATP to AMP [4]. The ubiquitin-protein makes a transfer to E2 via the E1 enzyme. The last step of the ubiquitylation reaction is finally catalyzed by E3 enzyme members. E3 interacts with E2 and the protein substrate; bring the ubiquitin transfer from E2 towards the substrate. As substrate becomes polyubiquitylated, with ZNF216 (upregulated by FoxO in muscle atrophy) recognition it is cropped to the proteasome systems following degradation during muscle atrophy. ZNF216-deficient mice are rather found resistant to muscle loss undergoing denervation. ZNF216 deficits in muscle cause accumulation of polyubiquitylated proteins [47]. Polyubiquitin protein chains can be detached through de-ubiquitylating enzymes [ubiquitin-specific processing proteases (USPs): USP14, USP19]. Atrogin-1 (specific ubiquitin ligase: MAFbx) regulates the t1/2 of the MyoD transcription factor and eIF3f (protein synthesis activator), which is a critical step in protein synthesis. The atrogin-1 knockdown avoids muscle loss during starvation in rodents [4, 48] while MuRF1 knockout (and not atrogin-1 knockout) are resilient against dexamethasone-provoke muscle atrophy [49]. Fbxo40 (ubiquitin ligase) regulates the t1/2 of IRS1, a necessary factor for IGF1/insulin signaling, while MuRF1 (specific ubiquitin ligase) regulates the t1/2 of several sarcomeric proteins [50].

2.6 Autophagy pathway

The discovery of autophagy in the year 1992 by Yoshinori Ohsumi changed the revolution of the machinery involved in orderly degradation and recycling of cellular components [51]. From then on enormous research has been done proving the importance of autophagy in eliminating invading pathogens, damaged organelles and toxic protein clearance in neurodegenerative disorders, attenuating neuroinflammation in dementia, Parkinson's, Alzheimer's [52, 53]. Furthermore, autophagy imparts a crucial role in the production of nutrients (amino acids, lipids, nucleic acids) during fasting [54]. The involvement of autophagy in muscle proteolysis during atrophy was recognized long back after the initial discovery of the mechanism of autophagy. Early studies significantly exhibit evidence that cathepsin L (lysosomal protease) was found with increased expression during muscle atrophy and lysosomal degradation was involved in protein breakdown in denervated muscles [55–57]. Molecular imaging techniques for visualization of autophagosome formation have improved the characterization of autophagy in atrophying muscles and normal cells. Multiple intracellular signaling mechanisms in diverse catabolic states and the role of atrogenes expression, protein degradation through the proteasome and autophagy pathways were studied.

The three major mechanisms involved in mammals for delivering autophagic cargo to lysosomes are macroautophagy, chaperone-mediated autophagy (CMA), and microautophagy [4]. The role of macroautophagy in muscle has been widely studied and microautophagy's role is yet to be discovered although some findings reveal the potential role of microautophagy for glycogen uptake within lysosomes at a time when macroautophagy is blocked [58, 59]. Macroautophagy generally is facilitated by activation of a regulatory complex (composed of Ambra1, Vps34, Vps15, Beclin 1, and Atg14) which further leads to recruit LC3 towards nascent autophagosome. Mitophagy (a selective form of macroautophagy) requires PINK1 and Bnip3 translocation factors. Scaffold protein p62 delivers the lysosomal degradation proteins (BAG3 and filamin) labeled by polyubiquitin chains to the autophagosome [60]. CMA majorly was studied for its crucial effects on neurodegenerative disorders, aging, and lysosomal storage diseases. In CMA, the damaged proteins due to excess ROS production express a definite amino acid sequence (KFERQ motif) which gets recognized by the Hsc70 chaperone and interacts with Lamp2a receptors delivers them to the lysosome [61]. Microautophagy engulfs small cytoplasmic portions into the lysosomes apart from breaking down glycogen in skeletal muscles. All three subtypes are involved contributing to protein degradation and remove organelle in skeletal muscles.

Autophagy is considered as a non-selective degradation pathway but with the advancement, in research, it has been shown that it can promote selective eradication of specific organelles (mitochondria) via mitophagy [62]. Skeletal muscles display the highest amount of vesicle formation when compared to other tissues during fasting conditions, confirming that in fasting conditions autophagosome formation is higher in glycolytic muscles rather than β-oxidative muscles [4]. Increased ROS production due to oxidative stress and impairment in the antioxidant defense systems is frequently seen in pathological conditions of muscle atrophy thus causing an imbalance in protein synthesis and degradation [63]. High ROS levels result in inhibition of insulin's actions acting as a putative mediator in the development of insulin resistance [63]. The increased oxidative stress in the muscle cells promotes the expression of autophagy proteins activating proteolytic pathways like calpain and ubiquitin-proteasome system. Dodd et al., 2010 conferred in their work that ROS might be the activator of the FOXO pathway and NF-kB in skeletal muscle atrophy [64].

The genes that regulate mitophagy are parkin, PINK1, Bnip3L, Bnip3 and inactivation in these genes may cause impaired mitochondria synthesis [65]. PINK1 assists the recruitment of parkin to mitochondria, parkin promotes mitophagy through ubiquitylation of mitochondrial membrane proteins recognized by p62 and adds autophagic vesicles for ubiquitylated mitochondrial proteins [66]. Autophagosome recruitment to mitochondria occurs as a result of Bnip3 and Bip3L binding to the LC3 domain [67]. Mitochondria network is remodeled during fasting and denervation via Bnip3 promoting autophagy. Inhibiting mitochondrial fission in mice was sufficient to prevent muscle atrophy during denervation providing significant insights in the importance of mitochondrial fission machinery, an impairment in basal mitophagy may lead to a disruption in the muscle homeostasis [16]. Besides mitophagy, nucleophagy may prove to be essential for the nuclear remodeling of muscle fibers [68].

3. Therapeutic targets and pharmacological interventions

The growing era of both synthetic and natural agents, characterized for targeting different aspects of NF-κB signaling. Targeting activators of NF-κB activation, such as TNF-α, monoclonal antibodies against TNF-α (infliximab) or decoy TNF receptors (e.g., etanercept), both drugs were found putting useful effects in the mdx model of DMD – decreasing myonecrosis and inhibits overall inflammation. The patients, who suffer from myositis, find with the raised expression of TNF-α in the muscle, anti-TNF therapies are not preferred. NEMO-binding domain (NBD) peptide interrupts the association of the IKK complex – which thwarts canonical NF-κB pathway activation [69]. NBD peptide in the mdx model of DMD decreases the macrophage infiltration into muscle and prevented overall membrane damage/lysis. Salicylates tend to inhibit NF-κB activation and ameliorate muscle damage. Natural compounds (curcumin, *Aloe vera*, berberine, apigenin, Quercetin, resve ratrol, 7,8-dihydroxyflavone, aspalathin, hesperidin, naringin, Epigallocatechin gallate, luteolin, rutin, Sulforaphane can target NF-κB signaling and harbors anti-NF-κB properties [70]. The use of antioxidants prevents inactivity-induced oxidative stress within skeletal muscles. Furthermore, antioxidants treatment to rodents could promote protein synthesis ad inhibits proteolysis. Numerous studies suggested that selected antioxidants such as vitamin E, Trolox and mitochondrial-targeted antioxidants, can lower inactivity-induced muscle atrophy in limb and respiratory muscles as well [71].

BDNF mimetic natural compound (7,8-dihydroxyflavone), chronically activate muscular TrkB modulates cellular energy expense and prohibit the development of excess body weight in female mice. These results reveal the molecular mechanism of targeting the TrkB receptor regulates cellular energy metabolism and improved motor activity [36, 72].

Certain evidence from *in vitro* studies concludes that Ferulic acid (polyphenolic compound), quercetin, luteolin, kaempferol, baicalin, rutin, naringin, and hesperidin regulates muscle fiber formation via activating Sirt1/AMPK signaling pathway. It activates Sirt1, which further activates LKB1 and AMPK. Sirt1 and AMPK congregate on enhancing the expression of PGC-1α and endorsing slow oxidative muscle fiber formation [72, 73]. Furthermore, Ex229 (a small molecule 991), PF-739, and MK-8722 activates AMPK within skeletal muscle [74].

Proteasome inhibitor such as MG132 significantly inhibits IκBα degradation and prevents NFκB activation *in vitro*. MG132 conserved muscle and its myofiber cross-sectional area via downregulating muscle-specific ubiquitin ligases: atrogin-1/MAFbx and MuRF-1 mRNA studied *in vivo* [75]. Furthermore, proteasome inhibitor Velcade (also known as PS-341 and bortezomib) directly inhibits the proteasome complex without directly impacting ubiquitination. This compound is usually orally active and is currently approved for treating multiple myeloma. Velcade utilization reduces skeletal muscle atrophy observed in denervated skeletal muscle in rats [76].

Myostatin and activin A antagonists: Myostatin, autocrine factor which normally confines muscle size. With growing evidence, increased generation of myostatin and its analog, activin A, contribute to several forms of atrophy. Inhibition of myostatin–activin A–GDF11 signaling is a hopeful therapy for multiple types of systemic wasting.

The SMA disease management utilizes a multidisciplinary and supportive approach, include neurologists (adult and pediatric), geneticists, respiratory physicians, gastroenterologists, orthopedic surgeons, palliative care physicians, rehabilitation specialists, and allied health services [2] (**Table 1**). Furthermore, **Table 2** describes the list of clinical trials with different approaches to treat SMA. There are

Complications	Assessments	Interventions
Respiratory	Cough effectiveness; respiratory muscle function tests; overnight oximetry; forced vital capacity (> 6 yrs)	Routine immunizations
		Annual influenza vaccination
	Overnight polysomnography if disordered breathing suspected; Acute respiratory infections	
		Airway clearance techniques and cough assistance- chest physiotherapy, postural drainage, mechanical or manual cough assistance
		Noninvasive ventilation
		Antibiotics intensified airway clearance
		Increased ventilation support
Gastrointestinal and nutritional	Feeding and swallowing assessment	Nutritional supplementation, modifying food consistency, optimal oral intake
		Nasogastric, nasojejunal or percutaneous gastronomy – as reduced oral intake is observed
		Nissen fundoplication
	Assess caloric intake	
	Assess for signs of reflux or aspiration	Hydration
	Assess for constipation	
Orthopedic and rehabilitation	Posture, mobility, function, Contractures, Scoliosis	Equipment to assist with mobility, self-care and function
		Physiotherapy, standing frames, Spinal Surgery
Psychological	Assess for depression or anxiety	Counseling, Antidepressants, Antianxiety drug managements

Table 1.
Current Management of Spinal Muscular Atrophy.

Study	Status	Type	Methods	Trial number	Sponsor
Gene Transfer Clinical Trial for Spinal Muscular Atrophy Type 1	Completed	Phase I, nonrandomized, open-label	Functional SMN gene is delivered intravenously using AAV9 The study involves three cohorts and escalating doses to evaluate safety and efficacy	NCT02122952	AveXis, Inc.
A Study to Assess the Efficacy and Safety of ISIS-SMNRx in Patients with Later-onset Spinal Muscular Atrophy	Completed	Phase III, RCT	ISIS-SMNRx is administered by intrathecal injections with small needle prick on the lower back	NCT02292537	Biogen
An Open-label Safety, Tolerability, and Dose-range Finding Study of ISIS-SMNRx in Patients with Spinal Muscular Atrophy	Completed	Phase I, nonrandomized, open-label	ISIS-SMNRx is administered as a single intrathecal injection	NCT01494701	Biogen
A Study to Assess the Safety and Pharmacokinetics of ISIS-SMNRx in Infants with Spinal Muscular Atrophy	Completed	Phase II, nonrandomized, open-label	Multiple doses of ISIS-SMNRx administered into the spinal fluid three times over the duration of the trial	NCT01839656	Biogen
An Open-label Safety, Tolerability and Dose-range Finding Study of Multiple Doses of ISIS-SMNRx in Patient with Spinal Muscular Atrophy (SMNRx-CS2)	Completed	Phase II, nonrandomized, open-label	Escalating doses of ISIS-SMNRx administered multiple times with intrathecal injections	NCT01703988	Biogen
An Open-label Safety and Tolerability Study of ISIS-SMNRx in Patients with Spinal Muscular Atrophy Who Previously Participated in ISIS 396443-CS1	Completed	Phase I, nonrandomized, open-label	Single dose of ISIS-SMNRx administered as a single intrathecal injection in patients who previously participated in ISIS 396443-CS1	NCT01780246	Biogen
An Open-label Safety and Tolerability Study of ISIS-SMNRx in Patients with Spinal Muscular Atrophy Who Previously Participated in ISIS SMNRx-CS2 or ISIS SMNRx-CS10	Completed	Phase I, nonrandomized, open-label	Multiple doses of ISIS-SMNRx administered as an intrathecal injection in patients who previously participated in ISIS 396443-CS2 or ISIS 396443-CS10	NCT02052791	Biogen
A study to assess the efficacy and safety of nusinersen (ISIS 396443) in infants with SMA (ENDEAR)	Terminated	Phase III, randomized, quadruple (participant, care provider,investigator, outcomes assessor)	ISIS-SMNRx* is administered by intrathecal injections with small needle prick on the lower back	NCT02193074	Biogen

Study	Status	Type	Methods	Trial number	Sponsor
A study for participants with SMA who previously participated in nusinersen (ISIS 396443) investigational studies (SHINE)	Active, Non recruiting	Phase III, nonrandomized, open-label	Administered by intrathecal (IT) injection to evaluate long term safety and tolerability	NCT02594124	Biogen
A Study of Multiple Doses of Nusinersen (ISIS 396443) Delivered to Infants With Genetically Diagnosed and Pre-symptomatic Spinal Muscular Atrophy (NURTURE).	Active, Non recruiting	Phase II, open-label	Intrathecal administration of multiple doses of nusinersen in infants with genetically diagnosed and pre-symptomatic SM	NCT02386553	Biogen
A study of RO6885247 in adult and pediatric patients with SMA (MOONFISH)	Terminated	Phase I, randomized double (participant, investigator)	Patients receive either RO6885247 or placebo in oral solution once daily for 12 weeks	NCT02240355	Hoffmann-La Roche
A study to investigate the safety, tolerability, pharmacokinetics and pharmacodynamics of RO7034067 (RG7916) given by mouth in healthy volunteer	Completed	Phase I, randomized, double (participant, investigator)	Oral administration of RO7034067 in healthy subjects to investigate safety, tolerability, pharmacokinetics and pharmacodynamics	NCT02633709	Hoffmann-La Roche
A study to investigate the safety, tolerability, pharmacokinetics, pharmacodynamics and efficacy of RO7034067 in participants with type 2 and 3 spinal SMA (Sunfish)	Active, Non recruiting	Phase II, III, randomized, double (participant, investigator)	Oral administration of RO7034067 in adult and pediatric patients with SMA2 and SMA3. The two-part study consists of an exploratory dose-finding part for 12 weeks and a confirmatory part for 24 months	NCT02908685	Hoffmann-La Roche
A study to investigate the safety, tolerability, pharmacokinetics, pharmacodynamics and efficacy of RO7034067 in infants with type 1 SMA (Firefish)	Active, Non recruiting	Phase II, III, nonrandomized, open-label	Oral administration of RO7034067 in infants with SMA1. The two-part study consists of an exploratory dose-finding part and a confirmatory part for 24 months at the dose selected in part 1	NCT02913482	Hoffmann-La Roche
A study of RO7034067 in adult and pediatric participants with SMA (Jewelfish)	Active, Non recruiting	Phase II, open- label	Oral administration of RO7034067 in adults and children with SMA2 and SMA3 previously treated with a SMN2targeting therapy	NCT03032172	Hoffmann-La Roche

DOI: http://dx.doi.org/10.5772/intechopen.95996

Study	Status	Type	Methods	Trial number	Sponsor
An open-label study of LMI070 in type 1 SMA	Active, Non recruiting	Phase I, II nonrandomized, open-label	Oral administration of LMI070 to investigate, the dose is safe for long term use or not	NCT02268552	Novartis Pharmaceuticals
Safety and efficacy of olesoxime (TRO19622) in patients with SMA aged 3–25 years	Completed	Phase II, randomized, quadruple (participant, care provider, investigator, outcomes assessor)	Administration of liquid suspension formulation (10 mg/kg) of olesoxime once a day with food at dinner to non-ambulant 3–25-year-old patients with SMA2 or SMA3	NCT01302600	Hoffmann-La Roche
A study to evaluate long term safety, tolerability, and effectiveness of olesoxime in participants with SMA	Completed	Phase II, open-label	Administration of 10 mg/kg suspension of olesoxime once a day either orally or via a nasogastric or gastrostomy tube in patients with SMA who participated in previous TRO19622 studies	NCT02628743	Hoffmann-La Roche
A study of CK-2127107 in patients with SMA	Completed	Phase II, randomized, triple (participant, investigator, treatment assessor)	Oral administration of multiple doses of CK-2127107 to ambulant and non-ambulant patients with SMA2, SMA3 and SMA4	NCT02644668	Cytokinetics
A Study to Assess the Safety and Tolerability of Nusinersen (ISIS 396443) in Participants With Spinal Muscular Atrophy (SMA). (EMBRACE)	Terminated	Phase II, randomized, quadruple (participant, care provider,investigator, outcomes assessor)	Multiple doses of Nusinersen administered as an intrathecal injection	NCT02462759	Biogen
An Active Treatment Study of SRK-015 in Patients with Type 2 or Type 3 Spinal Muscular Atrophy (TOPAZ)	Active, Non recruiting	Phase I, nonrandomized, open-label	Administration of SRK-015 intravenous infusion in SMA Type 2 and Type 3 in pediatric and adult patients, to investigate the safety and efficacy	NCT03921528	Scholar Rock,Inc.

Based on trials listed in https://www.clinicaltrials.gov/ and http://www.curesma.org/.

Table 2.
Clinical trials list with different approaches to treat Spinal Muscular atrophy.

Drugs	Disease	Route of Delivery	Outcomes	References
ActRIIB decoy	Lung and Bowel cancer	Subcutaneous injection	Reversed skeletal and cardiac muscle wasting and prolonged survival	[79]
Myostatin-specific antibody	Lung cancer	Subcutaneous injection	Inhibited muscle wasting and improved muscle function	[80]
Myostatin-specific peptibody	Kidney failure	Subcutaneous injection	Prevented Muscle wasting	[81]
JA-16 (myostatin-specific antibody)	Cardiac failure	Intraperitoneal Injection	Inhibited Muscle wasting	[82]
Myostatin-specific antibody	Disuse (hindlimb immobilization in plaster cast	Subcutaneous injection	Inhibited muscle wasting	[83]
Myostatin-specific antibody	Sarcopenia	Subcutaneous injection	Inhibited muscle wasting	[83]
STAT3 small-molecule inhibitor (C188–9)	Kidney failure	Subcutaneous injection	Inhibited muscle wasting	[84]

Table 3.
Studies of myostatin–activin pathway inhibitors in rodents.

Drug/target	Disease Process	Trial details	Outcomes	Ref. or Clinical Trials.gov.identifier
TNF-α				
Etanercept (TNFα ligand bound to Fc-IgG1	Cancer	IV administration RCT	No inhibition of muscle wasting	[85]
Infliximab (TNF-α specific mAb)	Non-small-cell lung cancer	IV administration RCT	Trial ceased early stages due to reduced patient quality life in infliximab-treated group	[86]
IL-6				
ALD518 (BMS-945429; IL-6 – specific mAb	Lung cancer	IV administration Phase I/II	No inhibition of muscle wasting	[87]
Myostatin/activin				
BYM338 (bimagrumab; ActRIIB-specific mAb)	Sarcopenia	IV administration RCT	In Progress	NCT01669174
	COPD	IV administration RCT	In Progress	NCT01601600

Drug/target	Disease Process	Trial details	Outcomes	Ref. or Clinical Trials.gov.identifier
	Cancer	IV administration RCT	In Progress	NCT01868685
	Mechanical ventilation	IV administration RCT	In Progress	NCT01433263
	Sporadic inclusion body myositis	IV administration RCT	In Progress	NCT01925209 (RESILIENT trial)
LY2495655 (myostatinspecificmAb)	Pancreatic cancer	IV administration Phase II	In Progress	NCT01505530
Ghrelin receptor				
Ghrelin	COPD	IV administration RCT	Improvement in quality of life but not physical activity	[88]
Anamorelin (growth hormone secretagogue receptor agonist)	Cancer	Oral administration RCT	Improved symptoms	[89]
	Non-small-cell lung cancer	Oral administration RCT	In Progress	NCT01387282
SUN11031 (ghrelin agonist)	COPD	Subcutaneous administration	Increased muscle mass but not function	NCT00698828
Androgen receptor				
Enobosarm	Aging	Oral administration Phase II	Increased muscle mass and function	[90]
	Cancer	Oral administration RCT	Increase muscle mass but not function	NCT01355484 and NCT01355497 (POWER trials); NCT00467844
MT-102 (SARM)	Non-small-cell lung cancer	Oral administration RCT	In Progress	ACT-ONE trial
GSK2849466 (SARM)	Healthy volunteers	Oral administration Phase I	Non-serious adverse events	NCT01696604
LGD-4033 (SARM)	Healthy volunteers	Oral administration Phase I	Non-serious adverse events	[91]

ActRIIB, activin A receptor, type IIB; COPD, chronic obstructive pulmonary disease; IgG1, immunoglobulin G1; IV, ntravenous; IL-6, interleukin-6; mAb, monoclonal antibody; RCT, randomized controlled trial; SARM, selective androgen receptor modulator

Table 4.
Clinical trials assessing treatments for muscle wasting.

some preclinical and clinical trials evaluating treatments for muscle wasting [77, 78] mentioned in **Tables 3** and **4**.

The Stem-cell-related therapies provide prominent therapeutic benefits in the reversal of condition in muscle atrophy thereby promoting muscle regeneration. Stem cell therapy (e.g., umbilical cord blood stem cell transplantation) showed helpful results for treating Duchenne muscular dystrophy (DMD). In the setting of a first-in-class approved therapy, progress in developing second generation and combination therapies will be requisite for novel approaches in trial design [92, 93]. Also, current new challenges are for developing therapies, together with difficulties access to treatment allied with complications, costs, and expertise which is required for intrathecal administration. Further efforts to ascertain optimal routes of drug delivery, body distribution, and limit safety therapeutic window must be essential.

4. Conclusion

Further, future directions are needed for developing novel safe, efficacious therapies with innovative therapeutic approaches for establishing a quality life in patients. The foremost challenge with developing therapies that grow muscle is preventing misuse for enhancing athletic performance, particularly anabolic steroids and growth hormones. Novel methods along with specific guidelines must be developed to monitor the numerous agents with potential remedial benefits of such therapies are likely to be considerable.

Acknowledgements

We gratefully acknowledge Department of Pharmaceuticals, Ministry of Chemical and Fertilizers, Government of India for providing technical support to this work.

Abbreviations

ALS	autophagy lysosomal system
AMPK	AMP activated protein kinase
BDNF	brain-derived neurotrophic factor
CMA	chaperone mediated autophagy
cPKC	protein kinase C
DMD	Duchenne muscular dystrophy
DRP1	dynamin related protein 1
FoxO	forkhead box transcription factors
IKKβ	IκB kinase
MFN	mitofusin
MAM	membrane associated-sarcoplasmic reticulum membranes
NF-κB	nuclear factor kappa-light-chain-enhancer of activated B cells
NGF	nerve growth factor
OPA1	optic atrophy 1
PGC-1α	proliferator-activated receptor gamma coactivator 1-alpha
ROS	reactive oxygen species
SBMA	spinal bulbar muscular atrophy
SMA	spinal Muscular Atrophy
SIRT1	silent information regulator/Sirtuin 1

DOI: http://dx.doi.org/10.5772/intechopen.95996

TrkB	tropomyosin-related kinase B receptor
TGF-β	transforming growth factor-β
TNF-α	tumor necrosis factor-α
TWEAK	TNF-like weak inducer of apoptosis
UPS	ubiquitin–proteasome system
VEGF	vascular endothelial growth factor

Author details

Mohit Kwatra*, Sahabuddin Ahmed, Samir Ranjan Panda, Vegi Ganga Modi Naidu and Nitika Gupta
Department of Pharmacology and Toxicology, National Institute of Pharmaceutical Education and Research (NIPER), Guwahati, Assam, India

*Address all correspondence to: mohitpharmacology@gmail.com

References

[1] McKinnell, I.W. and M.A. Rudnicki, Molecular Mechanisms of Muscle Atrophy. Cell, 2004. 119(7): p. 907-910.

[2] Farrar, M.A., et al., Emerging therapies and challenges in spinal muscular atrophy. Ann Neurol, 2017. 81(3): p. 355-368.

[3] van Helvoort, H.A., et al., Six-minute walking-induced systemic inflammation and oxidative stress in muscle-wasted COPD patients. Chest, 2007. 131(2): p. 439-45.

[4] Bonaldo, P. and M. Sandri, Cellular and molecular mechanisms of muscle atrophy. Dis Model Mech, 2013. 6(1): p. 25-39.

[5] Costamagna, D., et al., Role of Inflammation in Muscle Homeostasis and Myogenesis. Mediators Inflamm, 2015. 2015: p. 805172.

[6] Zhao, J., et al., Coordinate activation of autophagy and the proteasome pathway by FoxO transcription factor. Autophagy, 2008. 4(3): p. 378-80.

[7] Peterson, J.M., N. Bakkar, and D.C. Guttridge, NF-κB signaling in skeletal muscle health and disease. Curr Top Dev Biol, 2011. 96: p. 85-119.

[8] Cai, D., et al., IKKbeta/NF-kappaB activation causes severe muscle wasting in mice. Cell, 2004. 119(2): p. 285-98.

[9] Judge, A.R., et al., Role for IkappaBalpha, but not c-Rel, in skeletal muscle atrophy. Am J Physiol Cell Physiol, 2007. 292(1): p. C372-82.

[10] Hunter, R.B. and S.C. Kandarian, Disruption of either the Nfkb1 or the Bcl3 gene inhibits skeletal muscle atrophy. J Clin Invest, 2004. 114(10): p. 1504-11.

[11] de Alvaro, C., et al., Tumor necrosis factor alpha produces insulin resistance in skeletal muscle by activation of inhibitor kappaB kinase in a p38 MAPK-dependent manner. J Biol Chem, 2004. 279(17): p. 17070-8.

[12] Mourkioti, F., et al., Targeted ablation of IKK2 improves skeletal muscle strength, maintains mass, and promotes regeneration. J Clin Invest, 2006. 116(11): p. 2945-54.

[13] Dogra, C., et al., TNF-related weak inducer of apoptosis (TWEAK) is a potent skeletal muscle-wasting cytokine. FASEB journal : official publication of the Federation of American Societies for Experimental Biology, 2007. 21(8): p. 1857-1869.

[14] Mittal, A., et al., The TWEAK-Fn14 system is a critical regulator of denervation-induced skeletal muscle atrophy in mice. J Cell Biol, 2010. 188(6): p. 833-49.

[15] Bhatnagar, S. and A. Kumar, The TWEAK-Fn14 system: breaking the silence of cytokine-induced skeletal muscle wasting. Curr Mol Med, 2012. 12(1): p. 3-13.

[16] Romanello, V., et al., Mitochondrial fission and remodelling contributes to muscle atrophy. Embo j, 2010. 29(10): p. 1774-85.

[17] Kang, C., D. Yeo, and L.L. Ji, Muscle immobilization activates mitophagy and disrupts mitochondrial dynamics in mice. Acta Physiol (Oxf), 2016. 218(3): p. 188-197.

[18] de Brito, O.M. and L. Scorrano, Mitofusin-2 regulates mitochondrial and endoplasmic reticulum morphology and tethering: the role of Ras. Mitochondrion, 2009. 9(3): p. 222-6.

[19] Glauser, L., et al., Parkin promotes the ubiquitination and degradation of the mitochondrial fusion factor

mitofusin 1. J Neurochem, 2011. 118(4): p. 636-45.

[20] Taguchi, N., et al., Mitotic phosphorylation of dynamin-related GTPase Drp1 participates in mitochondrial fission. J Biol Chem, 2007. 282(15): p. 11521-9.

[21] Chou, C.H., et al., GSK3beta-mediated Drp1 phosphorylation induced elongated mitochondrial morphology against oxidative stress. PLoS One, 2012. 7(11): p. e49112.

[22] Vainshtein, A., et al., PGC-1α modulates denervation-induced mitophagy in skeletal muscle. Skelet Muscle, 2015. 5: p. 9.

[23] Cannavino, J., et al., The role of alterations in mitochondrial dynamics and PGC-1α over-expression in fast muscle atrophy following hindlimb unloading. J Physiol, 2015. 593(8): p. 1981-95.

[24] Hyatt, H., et al., Mitochondrial dysfunction induces muscle atrophy during prolonged inactivity: A review of the causes and effects. Arch BiochemBiophys, 2019. 662: p. 49-60.

[25] Sakuma, K. and A. Yamaguchi, The recent understanding of the neurotrophin's role in skeletal muscle adaptation. J Biomed Biotechnol, 2011. 2011: p. 201696.

[26] Ahmed, S., et al., Potential role of TrkB agonist in neuronal survival by promoting CREB/BDNF and PI3K/Akt signaling in vitro and in vivo model of 3-nitropropionic acid (3-NP)-induced neuronal death. Apoptosis, 2020.

[27] Pandey, S.N., et al., 7,8-Dihydroxyflavone alleviated the high-fat diet and alcohol-induced memory impairment: behavioral, biochemical and molecular evidence. Psychopharmacology (Berl), 2020. 237(6): p. 1827-1840.

[28] Dorsey, S.G., et al., Genetic deletion of trkB.T1 increases neuromuscular function. Am J Physiol Cell Physiol, 2012. 302(1): p. C141-53.

[29] Hurtado, E., et al., Muscle Contraction Regulates BDNF/TrkB Signaling to Modulate Synaptic Function through Presynaptic cPKCα and cPKCβI. Frontiers in Molecular Neuroscience, 2017. 10(147).

[30] Santafé, M.M., et al., Muscarinic autoreceptors modulate transmitter release through protein kinase C and protein kinase A in the rat motor nerve terminal. Eur J Neurosci, 2006. 23(8): p. 2048-56.

[31] Hurtado, E., et al., Muscle Contraction Regulates BDNF/TrkB Signaling to Modulate Synaptic Function through Presynaptic cPKCα and cPKCβI. Front Mol Neurosci, 2017. 10: p. 147.

[32] Ono, M., et al., Brain-derived neurotrophic factor reduces blood glucose level in obese diabetic mice but not in normal mice. BiochemBiophys Res Commun, 1997. 238(2): p. 633-7.

[33] Avila, A.M., et al., Trichostatin A increases SMN expression and survival in a mouse model of spinal muscular atrophy. J Clin Invest, 2007. 117(3): p. 659-71.

[34] McGee, S.L. and M. Hargreaves, Exercise and myocyte enhancer factor 2 regulation in human skeletal muscle. Diabetes, 2004. 53(5): p. 1208-14.

[35] Matthews, V.B., et al., Brain-derived neurotrophic factor is produced by skeletal muscle cells in response to contraction and enhances fat oxidation via activation of AMP-activated protein kinase. Diabetologia, 2009. 52(7): p. 1409-18.

[36] Chan, C.B., et al., Activation of muscular TrkB by its small molecular

agonist 7,8-dihydroxyflavone sex-dependently regulates energy metabolism in diet-induced obese mice. Chem Biol, 2015. 22(3): p. 355-68.

[37] Halievski, K., et al., Androgen-dependent loss of muscle BDNF mRNA in two mouse models of SBMA. Exp Neurol, 2015. 269: p. 224-32.

[38] Rodgers, J.T., et al., Nutrient control of glucose homeostasis through a complex of PGC-1alpha and SIRT1. Nature, 2005. 434(7029): p. 113-8.

[39] Brunet, A., et al., Stress-dependent regulation of FOXO transcription factors by the SIRT1 deacetylase. Science, 2004. 303(5666): p. 2011-5.

[40] Fulco, M., et al., Glucose restriction inhibits skeletal myoblast differentiation by activating SIRT1 through AMPK-mediated regulation of Nampt. Dev Cell, 2008. 14(5): p. 661-73.

[41] Costford, S.R., et al., Skeletal muscle NAMPT is induced by exercise in humans. Am J Physiol Endocrinol Metab, 2010. 298(1): p. E117-26.

[42] Sturrock, A., et al., Nox4 mediates TGF-beta1-induced retinoblastoma protein phosphorylation, proliferation, and hypertrophy in human airway smooth muscle cells. Am J Physiol Lung Cell Mol Physiol, 2007. 292(6): p. L1543-55.

[43] Rodgers, J.T., et al., Metabolic adaptations through the PGC-1 alpha and SIRT1 pathways. FEBS Lett, 2008. 582(1): p. 46-53.

[44] Kuno, A. and Y. Horio, SIRT1: A Novel Target for the Treatment of Muscular Dystrophies. Oxid Med Cell Longev, 2016. 2016: p. 6714686.

[45] Rasbach, K.A., et al., PGC-1alpha regulates a HIF2alpha-dependent switch in skeletal muscle fiber types. Proc Natl Acad Sci U S A, 2010. 107(50): p. 21866-71.

[46] Lee, D. and A.L. Goldberg, SIRT1 protein, by blocking the activities of transcription factors FoxO1 and FoxO3, inhibits muscle atrophy and promotes muscle growth. J Biol Chem, 2013. 288(42): p. 30515-26.

[47] Hishiya, A., et al., A novel ubiquitin-binding protein ZNF216 functioning in muscle atrophy. Embo j, 2006. 25(3): p. 554-64.

[48] Cong, H., et al., Inhibition of atrogin-1/MAFbx expression by adenovirus-delivered small hairpin RNAs attenuates muscle atrophy in fasting mice. Hum Gene Ther, 2011. 22(3): p. 313-24.

[49] Baehr, L.M., J.D. Furlow, and S.C. Bodine, Muscle sparing in muscle RING finger 1 null mice: response to synthetic glucocorticoids. J Physiol, 2011. 589(Pt 19): p. 4759-76.

[50] Shi, J., et al., The SCF-Fbxo40 complex induces IRS1 ubiquitination in skeletal muscle, limiting IGF1 signaling. Dev Cell, 2011. 21(5): p. 835-47.

[51] Ohsumi, Y., Yoshinori Ohsumi: autophagy from beginning to end. Interview by Caitlin Sedwick. J Cell Biol, 2012. 197(2): p. 164-5.

[52] Fougeray, S. and N. Pallet, Mechanisms and biological functions of autophagy in diseased and ageing kidneys. Nat Rev Nephrol, 2015. 11(1): p. 34-45.

[53] Ghavami, S., et al., Autophagy and apoptosis dysfunction in neurodegenerative disorders. Prog Neurobiol, 2014. 112: p. 24-49.

[54] Singh, R., Autophagy in the control of food intake. Adipocyte, 2012. 1(2): p. 75-79.

[55] Furuno, K., M.N. Goodman, and A.L. Goldberg, Role of different proteolytic systems in the degradation

of muscle proteins during denervation atrophy. J Biol Chem, 1990. 265(15): p. 8550-7.

[56] Deval, C., et al., Identification of cathepsin L as a differentially expressed message associated with skeletal muscle wasting. Biochem J, 2001. 360(Pt 1): p. 143-50.

[57] Schiaffino, S. and V. Hanzlíková, Studies on the effect of denervation in developing muscle. II. The lysosomal system. J Ultrastruct Res, 1972. 39(1): p. 1-14.

[58] Raben, N., et al., Suppression of autophagy in skeletal muscle uncovers the accumulation of ubiquitinated proteins and their potential role in muscle damage in Pompe disease. Hum Mol Genet, 2008. 17(24): p. 3897-908.

[59] Takikita, S., et al., Fiber type conversion by PGC-1α activates lysosomal and autophagosomal biogenesis in both unaffected and Pompe skeletal muscle. PLoS One, 2010. 5(12): p. e15239.

[60] Galluzzi, L., et al., Molecular definitions of autophagy and related processes. Embo j, 2017. 36(13): p. 1811-1836.

[61] Kon, M. and A.M. Cuervo, Chaperone-mediated autophagy in health and disease. FEBS Lett, 2010. 584(7): p. 1399-404.

[62] Ding, W.X. and X.M. Yin, Mitophagy: mechanisms, pathophysiological roles, and analysis. Biol Chem, 2012. 393(7): p. 547-64.

[63] Powers, S.K., A.N. Kavazis, and J.M. McClung, Oxidative stress and disuse muscle atrophy. J Appl Physiol (1985), 2007. 102(6): p. 2389-97.

[64] Dodd, S.L., et al., Ros-mediated activation of NF-kappaB and Foxo during muscle disuse. Muscle Nerve, 2010. 41(1): p. 110-3.

[65] Hara, T., et al., Suppression of basal autophagy in neural cells causes neurodegenerative disease in mice. Nature, 2006. 441(7095): p. 885-9.

[66] Narendra, D.P. and R.J. Youle, Targeting mitochondrial dysfunction: role for PINK1 and Parkin in mitochondrial quality control. Antioxid Redox Signal, 2011. 14(10): p. 1929-38.

[67] Hanna, R.A., et al., Microtubule-associated protein 1 light chain 3 (LC3) interacts with Bnip3 protein to selectively remove endoplasmic reticulum and mitochondria via autophagy. J Biol Chem, 2012. 287(23): p. 19094-104.

[68] Park, Y.E., et al., Autophagic degradation of nuclear components in mammalian cells. Autophagy, 2009. 5(6): p. 795-804.

[69] Li, H., S. Malhotra, and A. Kumar, Nuclear factor-kappa B signaling in skeletal muscle atrophy. J Mol Med (Berl), 2008. 86(10): p. 1113-26.

[70] Rondanelli, M., et al., A Systematic Review on the Effects of Botanicals on Skeletal Muscle Health in Order to Prevent Sarcopenia. Evidence-Based Complementary and Alternative Medicine, 2016. 2016: p. 5970367.

[71] Powers, S.K., Can antioxidants protect against disuse muscle atrophy? Sports Med, 2014. 44 Suppl 2(Suppl 2): p. S155-65.

[72] Korkmaz, O.T., et al., 7,8-Dihydroxyflavone improves motor performance and enhances lower motor neuronal survival in a mouse model of amyotrophic lateral sclerosis. Neurosci Lett, 2014. 566: p. 286-91.

[73] Chen, X., et al., Ferulic acid regulates muscle fiber type formation through the Sirt1/AMPK signaling pathway. Food & Function, 2019. 10(1): p. 259-265.

[74] Olivier, S., M. Foretz, and B. Viollet, Promise and challenges for direct small molecule AMPK activators. BiochemPharmacol, 2018. 153: p. 147-158.

[75] Caron, A.Z., et al., The proteasome inhibitor MG132 reduces immobilization-induced skeletal muscle atrophy in mice. BMC MusculoskeletDisord, 2011. 12: p. 185.

[76] Beehler, B.C., et al., Reduction of Skeletal Muscle Atrophy by a Proteasome Inhibitor in a Rat Model of Denervation. Experimental Biology and Medicine, 2006. 231(3): p. 335-341.

[77] Furrer, R. and C. Handschin, Muscle Wasting Diseases: Novel Targets and Treatments. Annu Rev PharmacolToxicol, 2019. 59: p. 315-339.

[78] Cohen, S., J.A. Nathan, and A.L. Goldberg, Muscle wasting in disease: molecular mechanisms and promising therapies. Nat Rev Drug Discov, 2015. 14(1): p. 58-74.

[79] Zhou, X., et al., Reversal of cancer cachexia and muscle wasting by ActRIIB antagonism leads to prolonged survival. Cell, 2010. 142(4): p. 531-43.

[80] Murphy, K.T., et al., Antibody-directed myostatin inhibition enhances muscle mass and function in tumor-bearing mice. Am J PhysiolRegulIntegr Comp Physiol, 2011. 301(3): p. R716-26.

[81] Zhang, L., et al., Pharmacological inhibition of myostatin suppresses systemic inflammation and muscle atrophy in mice with chronic kidney disease. Faseb j, 2011. 25(5): p. 1653-63.

[82] Heineke, J., et al., Genetic deletion of myostatin from the heart prevents skeletal muscle atrophy in heart failure. Circulation, 2010. 121(3): p. 419-25.

[83] Murphy, K.T., et al., Acute antibody-directed myostatin inhibition attenuates disuse muscle atrophy and weakness in mice. J Appl Physiol (1985), 2011. 110(4): p. 1065-72.

[84] Zhang, L., et al., Stat3 activation links a C/EBPδ to myostatin pathway to stimulate loss of muscle mass. Cell Metab, 2013. 18(3): p. 368-79.

[85] Jatoi, A., et al., A placebo-controlled double blind trial of etanercept for the cancer anorexia/weight loss syndrome: results from N00C1 from the North Central Cancer Treatment Group. Cancer, 2007. 110(6): p. 1396-403.

[86] Jatoi, A., et al., A placebo-controlled, double-blind trial of infliximab for cancer-associated weight loss in elderly and/or poor performance non-small cell lung cancer patients (N01C9). Lung Cancer, 2010. 68(2): p. 234-9.

[87] Bayliss, T.J., et al., A humanized anti-IL-6 antibody (ALD518) in non-small cell lung cancer. Expert Opin Biol Ther, 2011. 11(12): p. 1663-8.

[88] Miki, K., et al., Ghrelin treatment of cachectic patients with chronic obstructive pulmonary disease: a multicenter, randomized, double-blind, placebo-controlled trial. PLoS One, 2012. 7(5): p. e35708.

[89] Garcia, J.M., J. Friend, and S. Allen, Therapeutic potential of anamorelin, a novel, oral ghrelin mimetic, in patients with cancer-related cachexia: a multicenter, randomized, double-blind, crossover, pilot study. Support Care Cancer, 2013. 21(1): p. 129-37.

[90] Dalton, J.T., et al., The selective androgen receptor modulator GTx-024 (enobosarm) improves lean body mass and physical function in healthy elderly men and postmenopausal women: results of a double-blind, placebo-controlled phase II trial. J Cachexia Sarcopenia Muscle, 2011. 2(3): p. 153-161.

[91] Basaria, S., et al., The safety, pharmacokinetics, and effects of LGD-4033, a novel nonsteroidal oral, selective androgen receptor modulator, in healthy young men. J GerontolA Biol Sci Med Sci, 2013. 68(1): p. 87-95.

[92] Fukada, S.I., The roles of muscle stem cells in muscle injury, atrophy and hypertrophy. J Biochem, 2018. 163(5): p. 353-358.

[93] Shadrach, J.L. and A.J. Wagers, Stem cells for skeletal muscle repair. Philos Trans R Soc Lond B Biol Sci, 2011. 366(1575): p. 2297-306.

Chapter 2

Skeletal Muscle Stem Cell Niche from Birth to Old Age

Madalina-Gabriela Barbu, Andreea-Elena Boboc, Lidia Filip, Oana-Larisa Bugnar, Dragos Cretoiu, Nicolae Suciu, Oana Daniela Toader, Sanda Maria Cretoiu and Silviu-Cristian Voinea

Abstract

Stem cells are defined as undifferentiated cells that are able to unlimitedly renew themselves within controlled conditions and to differentiate into a multitude of mature cell types. Skeletal muscle stem cells, represented predominantly by satellite cells, show a variable capability of self-renewal and myogenic differentiation. They were found to be involved not only in the growth of myofibers during neonatal and juvenile life but also in the regeneration of skeletal muscles after an injury. The microenvironment in which stem cells are nourished and maintained dormant preceding division and differentiation is known as "niche." The niche consists of myofibers, which are believed to modulate the active/inactive state of the stem cells, extracellular matrix, neural networks, blood vessels, and a multitude of soluble molecules. It was observed that changes in the composition of the niche have an impact on the stem cell functions and hierarchy. Furthermore, it seems that its layout is variable throughout the entire life, translating into a decrease in the regenerative capacity of satellite cells in aged tissues. The scope of this chapter is to provide a detailed view of the changes that occur in the skeletal stem cell niche during life and to analyze their implications on tissue regeneration. Future studies should focus on developing new therapeutic tools for diseases involving muscle atrophy.

Keywords: stem cells, niche, skeletal, aging, regeneration, muscle fibers

1. Introduction

Being crucial for the survival, the striated muscle tissue that forms skeletal muscles takes up to 40% of the human body weight and is responsible for locomotion, maintaining the posture of the body, breathing, swallowing, micturition, and defecation [1, 2]. Furthermore, skeletal muscles were found to present endocrine and paracrine functions through the secretion of myokines, as well as thermogenesis abilities [3]. Each muscle comprises a multitude of myofibers that organize themselves into fascicles by wrapping with a layer of connective tissue known as perimysium [4]. Myofibers are long, cylindrical multinucleated cells that are individually enveloped in another layer of connected tissue called endomysium [4]. The myofibers provide skeletal muscles with contractile abilities and are formed in the prenatal life by the fusion of a number of cell progenitors known as myoblasts [2].

While the myofibers enable the muscle to contract and exert its functions, there are other types of cells, known as skeletal muscle stem cells that were proved to be responsible for muscle regeneration after injury [5]. Stem cells were defined as undifferentiated cells that present self-renewal abilities when proper stimuli exist and can generate various mature cell types through differentiation [6]. The environment in which stem cells are found is known as "niche" and its changes in composition were found to consequently influence their behavior [1]. Previous research regarding the characteristics of the niche found that its composition is highly heterogenic, varying not only with age, but also with the demands of the body [7]. In general, the muscular niche comprises an extracellular matrix known as the basal lamina, various interstitial cells such as fibroblasts and adipocytes, blood vessels, neural fibers, and a multitude of growth factors and signaling molecules [5].

Satellite cells, which are the most frequent stem cells found in the skeletal muscles, were first observed on the electron microscope by Alexander Mauro over 50 years ago [8]. They were given this name due to their sublaminar position and their close connection to myofibers [2]. Following their discovery, numerous studies were conducted in order to uncover the role they play in muscle repair and regeneration and how the stem cell niche is modulating their behavior [2]. In addition to their involvement in muscle repair, recent studies suggest that the skeletal muscle stem cells might even play a secondary role in bone regeneration [9]. Although satellite cells are the most frequent and easiest to study, other stem cell populations residing either in the skeletal muscle, or in other tissues, were found to possess variable muscle regenerative abilities [10]. Satellite cell properties as well as the different types of muscle progenitors will be described in detail in this chapter.

Studies showed that the number of myofibers does not change during the first stages of life and that the growth of the muscular system is obtained through the fusion of satellite cells with myofibers, resulting in an increase in size of the latter [2]. After the physiological growth of the organism stops, the skeletal stem cells are maintained in an inactivated state by various factors in the stem cell niche until they are needed for muscle repair or to participate in the daily muscle turnover [11].

The satellite cells are activated by growth stimuli or by the physical trauma located in the muscle, leading them to enter the mitotic phase and start to divide into myoblasts, which through differentiation will be able to fuse among themselves and with other myofibers and repair the damaged muscle [12, 13]. In addition, satellite cells can expand their stem cell pool through asymmetric division, thus demonstrating their self-renewal abilities and ensuring the continuance of the muscle regeneration process [12]. However, with aging and also in various degenerative muscle diseases, the regenerative abilities of satellite cells diminish, leading to muscle atrophy and the replacement of muscle fibers with connective tissue [7, 14]. These changes were attributed to a multitude of changes in the composition of the stem cell niche that occur during life, which will be further described in this chapter [7, 14].

The alteration of the skeletal stem cell niche and thus of satellite cell functions can be seen not only in aged muscle but also in a multitude of degenerative diseases. One example is Duchenne muscular dystrophy (DMD), a genetic disorder with no existing curative treatment in which a specific gene mutation causes the synthesis of an altered protein known as dystrophin, thus leading to progressive muscle degeneration and fibrosis which will result in loss of ambulation and cardiorespiratory insufficiency [15]. Dystrophin is known to be responsible for the basal lamina-myofibers connection; however, recent studies showed that it is also involved in the modulation of muscle stem cell division [13]. Additional research is needed in order to fully understand how satellite cells and their niches are affected by DMD.

It is crucial to understand all the pathways that are involved in the functioning of the skeletal stem cell niche and the way they are altered with the aging of the human body in order to be able to develop new treatment strategies for muscle degenerative diseases and maybe delay the effects that time has on the muscular system. Extensive research has been made in the field of regenerative medicine, making the idea of bioengineered muscle regeneration increasingly plausible. However, there are still many unanswered questions that prevent the applications of satellite cell's regenerative and self-renewal abilities to reach their full potential.

2. The skeletal muscle stem cell niche: structure and roles

The stem cell niche concept was first described in 1978 by Schofield, as an explanation to a series of experimental findings focusing on hematopoiesis and the bone marrow cells, which outlined notions concerning the anatomic site of reproduction, sustenance, and differentiation of the stem cells [16–18]. According to this theory, the niche represents a versatile environment, where the states change cyclically, in order to either support the quiescence of the stem cells or to activate them, according to the local or systemic stimuli [14]. Each type of tissue has a specific support system characterized by distinct cellular components; some of the most studied ones belonging to sites which present a high turnover rate such as the skin, with the matrix stem cells and the dermal papilla, the gut with the crypt stem cells and the mesenchymal and Paneth cells, or the hematopoietic stem cell niche and osteoblasts [14, 19, 20].

The skeletal muscle stem cell niche is also an example of a highly designated niche, consisting not only of specialized stem cells such as the satellite cells, but also of a complex milieu of elements ranging from the neural-vascular framework and surrounding cells to the extracellular matrix and diverse soluble molecules [2, 21]. In this chapter, we discuss in detail the cellular structure of the niche and the various roles that every type of constituent plays in the muscle behavior in regards to growth, maintenance, and regeneration [22].

2.1 Satellite cells and other muscle progenitors

During embryogenesis, the paraxial segmental mesoderm gives rise to the somites, which subsequently divide into the dermomyotome, which further generates the skeletal muscle of the body and limbs as well as the overlying derma, and the sclerotome, which contributes to the cartilage and bone formation of the spine and rib cage [10, 23, 24]. In the first stages of muscle development, a primary myotome is formed by delamination of muscle progenitor cells, expressing MYf5 and Mrf4, from the epithelial dermomyotome [25]. Subsequently, another subtype of muscle progenitors that express Pax7 and Pax3 migrate from the central dermomyotome toward the primary myotome, where some contribute to the further differentiation and growth and of the muscle, while others maintain a continuous pool of muscle progenitors that represent the largest reservoir of adult satellite cells for the muscles of the trunk and limbs [26, 27]. During the last decades, extensive research has been conducted in order to determine other types of non-somitic muscle stem progenitors, concluding that the embryonic dorsal aorta [28] can also serve as origin for the stem cells, along with various cells that exhibit myogenic potential such as the bone marrow stem cells [29, 30], pericytes [31], mesangioblasts [32], specific side population cells [33], and interstitial and mesenchymal cells [34, 35].

The first description of a satellite cell was made in 1961, when Katz and Mauro discovered a mononucleated cell positioned at the outer edge of the muscle fiber, while studying the muscle tissue in frogs and rats with the help of electron microscopy [8, 36]. Using the same imaging technique, it was established not only the cell's location between the basal lamina and the exterior plasma membrane of the myocyte, but also the morphological features: a small nucleus with elevated levels of heterochromatin, an abundant cytoplasm, and scarce organelles [37]. Since their discovery, extensive efforts have been made in order to demonstrate the stem cell characteristics and to identify the role they play in muscle growth and regeneration. In this regard, [3H]thymidine labeling and tracing experiments in regenerating or growing muscle proved that satellite cells contribute to this process by yielding myonuclei to emerging myofibers [38, 39]. To strengthen this evidence, in vitro cultures of isolated myofibers and their adjacent satellite cells showed that renewed myotubes arise from the satellite cell-derived myoblasts clonal expansion and fusion, demonstrating thus the stem cell's regenerative capacity [40–44].

Regeneration of the muscle tissue is a complex process that can be induced by either disease, injury, or exercise, involving a series of events like cellular degeneration, inflammation, further stem cell activation, and differentiation, followed by maturation and remodeling of the new fibers and the surrounding environment [45–47]. Activation of the satellite cells implies transitioning from the quiescent phase to a mitotic phase, event in which a series of signaling pathways and molecular elements, such as notch signaling pathway and map kinase phosphorylation process by the hepatocyte growth factor activation (HGF) and fibroblast growth factor 2 (FGF2), among others, participate [48–52]. Upon activation, satellite cells start expressing MyoD, a transcription factor promoting genes involved in the progression of the cell cycle, and along with preexisting expression of Pax7, M-cadherin, and Myf5, they start dividing [53, 54]. The differentiation process of the newly created myoblasts is governed by the Wnt signaling pathway, FGF, myostatin, an important regulator of muscle stem cell proliferation [55–57], which works together with myogenin and MyoD to generate multinucleated myofibers [58–60].

Apart from the regenerative capacity, satellite cells possess the ability to renew themselves, generating thus a continuous pool of stem cells. This theory of self-renewal was first stipulated in the pulse-chase experiments of Moss and Leblond, being further supported by the studies of other lineages such as the skin and gut that showed similarities between the transit amplifying cells and satellite cells [38, 61–63]. Another study focusing on transplanted myofibers in a myopathic mouse model found that a new population of satellite cells was generated after the resident muscle stem cells were inactivated by radiation, demonstrating thus the self-regenerating ability of the satellite cells [64]. As mentioned before, in restoring muscle tissue, satellite cells undergo a transition from a quiescent state to an activated state. Recent studies have demonstrated that the reverse process can also take place, as the activated satellite cells can exit the cell cycle and reenter the quiescent state, replenishing thus the progenitor pool [65–67], still, further research is required in order to elucidate the exact mechanisms of the self-renewal process.

Extensive research concluded that the satellite cells do not represent the only type of cell capable of muscle regeneration; several other cells exhibiting similar characteristics of which bone marrow stem cells [29, 30], pericytes [31], mesangioblasts [32] and specific side population cells [33] are some of the most studied ones. In this regard, strong evidence coming from lineage experiments indicated that bone marrow-derived stem cells, when administered intravenously or intramuscularly in irradiated mice, have the capacity to generate myofibers and to restore the satellite cell pool [68]. Following a study regarding the GFP-labeled bone marrow transplantation into mice, LaBarge and Blau et al. also concluded that bone marrow stem cells display myogenic potential by reconstructing the stem cell niche [68]. Recent studies suggest that pericytes, the contractile cells responsible for the regulation of capillary blood flow, exhibit a multipotent trait, allowing them to differentiate not only toward the skeletal bone and adipose tissue precursors but also into skeletal stem cells [69–71]. Prototype experiments involving pericyte transplantation in mice with dystrophic muscles proved that pericytes may represent a promising candidate for future treatments for similar affliction in humans due to their myogenic potential [31, 72].

2.2 Satellite cell cellular and acellular environment

The skeletal muscle stem cell niche is the biologic environment of the satellite cells and other muscle progenitor cells where biochemical and biophysical factors sustain cellular processes such as quiescence, self-renewal, multiplication and differentiation, necessary for maintenance, and repair of the muscle. Apart from stem cells and myofibers, the niche is a home to a variety of other cellular and acellular components ranging from the basal lamina, connective tissue, nerves, vessels, extracellular matrix, or immune cells that together design the optimal conditions to assist the transition through the various processes of the niche.

In this respect, one of the most intimate structures within the niche is the basal lamina, a network of extracellular matrix composed of collagen IV, laminin α2, fibronectin, and tenascin, linked together through a glycoprotein core of heparan sulfate [18, 73, 74]. This structure enables not only the anatomical sustenance of the myofibers through integrin linkage but also accumulations of growth factors such as FGF, HGF, VEGF, and TGFβ1 [75–77]. Several studies concluded that the loss or deficiency of laminin α2 impacts the muscle stem niche quiescence by reducing the number of stem cells during development, as well as increased myogenin expression, inhibiting proper differentiation [78, 79].

Another major component of the niche environment is represented by the interstitial cells, of which the most abundant types are the fibroblasts and the adipocytes. Both of these types of cells increase in number due to the transdifferentiating potential of the myoblasts and satellite cells showed by in vitro studies [80, 81], supporting the hypothesis that the muscle is able to sustain a balanced environment during regenerative processes. Nevertheless, surplus in number regarding adipocytes and excess connective tissue produced by the fibroblasts have been thoroughly linked to conditions, such as aging or muscular dystrophy [82–84].

The vascular network is one of the main nourishment suppliers for the stem cell muscle niche, playing an important role not only in angiogenesis but also in myogenesis. It has been shown that these two processes emerge simultaneously during muscle regeneration, the most important factors involved in this event being represented by VEGF, IGF-I, PDGF, and HGF [85]. VEGF has been observed to stimulate not only angiogenesis but also cell migration and differentiation, myofiber hypertrophy to prevent apoptosis [86–88].

Several studies have observed that stem cells tend to group around the neuromuscular junction, suggesting that the motor neurons interact with the niche during specific times. Denervation studies portrayed that the modifications in membrane potential, ion channel conductance, and distribution of acetylcholine receptors lead to the remodeling of the niche composition, following the activation of the muscle stem cells [89]. A combination between the absence of neurotrophic factors and a prolonged state of loss in neural communication has been also proved to lead to structural alterations, more specifically to myofiber atrophy [90].

This dynamic environment can be also influenced by a number of systemic factors, some of them being represented by immune cells and inflammation, androgens or nitric oxide [2]. Upon injury, satellite cells release the proinflammatory cytokines that promote immune cell migration to the muscle that in turn help the stem cells to detach from the basal lamina through a series of diffusible molecules, in order for them to further proliferate, differentiate, and repair the muscle in regards to muscle [91]. Androgens seem to impact the satellite cell nice by stimulating the stem cell activation and proliferation, while nitric oxide has been shown to provide a protective effect against fibrosis [92, 93].

3. Alterations of the skeletal stem cell niche during aging

Satellite cells, known as muscle specific stem cells, take the responsibility of generating new muscle fibers as a response to injury in the adult human body. However, the regenerative abilities of an aged muscle are significantly reduced, while the susceptibility of developing age-related pathologies is increased [14]. In order to better understand the mechanisms that contribute to declining stem cell function with age, it is important to firstly identify the cell-extrinsic and cell-intrinsic factors that have an influence on stem cell activity. Conditions within the niche are extremely important in order to maintain stem cell activity, and they need to be conducive to maintaining stem cell quiescence in the absence of any external activating cues while also promoting proliferation, maturation, and ensuring the self-renewal of the stem cell pool. Thus, the niche represents an inherently dynamic environment, which switches between the quiescent and the activated niche as a response to local and systemic influences. Any perturbation between the cell resident in the immediate vicinity and in direct contact with the stem cell is predicted to alter stem cell function [94]. Some previous research was focused on describing the characteristics of satellite cells residing in aged muscle, thus providing critical information on the transformations that occur with the passing of time. One study conducted on old mice revealed that the nuclear-cytoplasmic ratio is significantly higher compared to other cytological features that are almost identical with the ones identified in younger mice [95]. During the aging process, satellite stem cells display a delayed response to activating stimuli and also have a reduced proliferative expansion due to the fact that some progenitors tend to adopt alternate lineages [80, 82, 96, 97]. Furthermore, satellite cells were described to have higher apoptosis rates in the aged muscles [98].

In aging muscles, due to the accumulation of toxic products derived from the degradation of connective tissue components, some essential functions of the basal lamina are compromised. Necrosis is the result of the cleavaged fibronectin and elastin products present in the connective tissue of aging mice [99]. Studies on aged muscle sections revealed the presence of extra lamina encroaching into the satellite cell-myofiber interspace and mononucleated cells completely enveloped by the basal lamina [95]. Although the functional consequences of this less intimate association of satellite cells with myofibers in aged muscles are still unknown, it is believed that this phenomenon can be correlated to the decreasing percent of satellite cells in the later stages of life [82].

Numerous studies were conducted focusing on the molecular mechanisms that underline satellite cell aging. Heterochronic satellite cells were transplanted from old mice into young specimens, indicating that the mechanisms that modulate the satellite cell regeneration potential may be cell-extrinsic. Furthermore, various changes were observed regarding the availability of Wnt, Notch, FGF, and TGF-β-superfamily ligands, and also in cytokine signaling through the JAK-STAT pathway. Moreover, the self-renewal defects may be cell-intrinsic, as satellite cell aging was associated with an increase in stress-induced p38-MAPK signaling and cellular senescence [100].

3.1 Niche composition and functions at birth and in the early life

Myogenesis is a well-controlled process in which the dermomyotome is formed from the dorsolateral side of the somite, and from there, the progenitor cells will differentiate in order to form multinucleated myofibers [24, 101, 102]. Even if it was thought to be an interrelation between the existence of multipotent cells and tissue development, a group of somatic stem cells was discovered both in mature and early post-natal skeletal muscle. These are believed to have important contribution in regeneration, homeostasis, and muscle growth [103].

The first remarks about a stem cell population that originate in skeletal muscle were made by Mauro and Katz in 1961 [8, 104]. They analyzed the muscle samples from frog and rat, and using electron microscopy for identification, they postulated that satellite stem cells are located in a particular place (between the basal lamina and the sarcolemma), and it represents an exclusive niche which preserves and regulates the survival and behavior of the stem cell [105]. Satellite cells express specific markers: Pax7 and Pax3 (paired box transcription factors) [106, 107], M-cadherin [108], FoxK (Forkhead box protein K) [109], NCAM (neural cell adhesion molecule) [110] c-Met (tyrosine-protein kinase Met) [111], VCAM-1 [112], CD34 [113], Syndecan 3, Syndecan 4 [114], Sox 8 and Sox 15 [115, 116], Integrin α7, Integrin β1 [117], caveolin-1 [118], CTR (Calcitonin receptor) [119], Emerin, Lamin A/C [120], Hairy [121], and Dystrophin [122].

During post-natal life, satellite cells are responsible for muscle growth and tissue regeneration under the action of appropriate stimuli. This role was confirmed by a study which analyzed transgenic mice without satellite stem cells. The mice revealed a significant deficiency in skeletal muscle mass, lower body weight, and smaller myofiber size [106]. An important decrease in the number of cells was observed, from 30% at birth to 5% at 2 months old. In the adult life period, the cell number remained constant [123]. Even if the implication of satellite cells in muscle regeneration has been well documented and described, their role in muscle growth during adult life still needs further studies [124].

3.2 Changes in niche composition throughout the time

Discovering the link between stem cells and their niches presents a great interest for the biology field. Although previous reports debating the caring relationship between stem cells and signaling molecules deployed by niche cells were published, the role of extra-cellular matrix (ECM) into the niche is still unclear. Previous studies highlighted that at activation, satellite cells are responsible for establishing the local reshaping of the ECM, and for the accumulation of laminin-α1 and laminin-α5 right into the basal lamina of the satellite cell niche. Moreover, genetic modification of laminin-α1, integrin-α6 signaling, or blocking matrix metalloproteinase activity were shown to prevent the cell capacity of expansion and self-renewal. Remodeling of the ECM favors dissemination and self-renewal, and could justify the effect of laminin-α1 containing supports on stem cells [5].

Stem cells competence decreases with age, and it is associated with chronic diseases in mammals. In diseased or aged muscles, myofibers are replaced by fat and fibrous tissues, while the remaining myofibers decrease in mass. During aging, not only the percent of satellite cells decreases, but also their expression levels of Pax7, consequently leading to a decrease in myogenicity and an increase in apoptosis [125].

4. Implications on muscular regeneration and disease

Skeletal muscles possess contractile properties that are crucial for vital functions of the body such as breathing, postural support, and movement while also participating in the systemic metabolism and thermogenesis due to their endocrine and paracrine functions [3]. Following actions that involve contraction and stretch, micro-lesions can occur in the plasma membrane of muscular cells or in the T-tubule organization, leading to the organization of specific proteins and lipids which form a repair-patch and seal the injury. However, during trauma or surgery numerous contusions, strains and laceration can occur, and, in these circumstances, myoblasts fuse between themselves or with adjacent myofibers and repair the damaged muscle. One important fact is that myoblasts can only fuse with non-lethally damaged muscle cells [126–128].

It is widely known that skeletal muscle has a remarkable capacity for regeneration, which places it second after the bone marrow. The main type of stem cells in charge of muscle regeneration is represented by satellite cells. Satellite cells are able to remain in a non-dividing state in the unharmed muscle and can be recognized by their α7 integrin and Pax7 expression. This specific population of cells gets triggered when muscle trauma occurs, thus activating the expression of MYF5 and MYOD and becoming fusion-competent myoblasts which will further fuse in order to give rise to new muscle fibers [8, 129–132]. During muscle injury, there are satellite cells that do not differentiate, with downregulated MYF5 and MYOD expression levels, which were described to replace the satellite cell population, ensuring the ability to respond to future muscle damages [2, 67, 133, 134].

Studies showed that alongside with satellite cells, there exist various populations of non-satellite cells, such as side populations, CD133 + cells, pericytes, and mesangioblasts (Mabs) that have myogenic abilities, contributing to regeneration and homeostasis maintenance [31, 135–138]. Their involvement in muscle regeneration was not firmly demonstrated and future studies are needed. The regenerative capacity of this cell category was demonstrated following some experiments on mice [135]. Side population cells were transplanted into mice suffering from a form of Duchenne muscular dystrophy, leading to an improvement in muscle function and a restoration of dystrophin expression levels [135]. Similar results were obtained by intraarterial or intramuscular injecting CD 133+ cells into scid/mdx mice [136, 139]. Two other populations of non-satellite cells are pericytes and Mabs, the latter were described to derive from pericytes [31]. Pericytes are involved in the in situ regeneration and muscle growth in early life [140]. Studies revealed that Mabs can take part in muscular regeneration after being engrafted or intraarterial injected in dogs and mice [137, 138]. Researchers discovered that the behavior of satellite cells could be highly influenced by surrounding cells, growth factors such as the vascular endothelial growth factor (VEGF), insulin-like growth factor (IGF)-1, fibroblast growth factor (FGF), cytokines, and neighboring cellular matrix [141]. For example, one study showed that satellite cells which have grown in vitro for a short period of time partially lost their myogenic capacity in contrast to freshly isolated satellite cells [129]. In order to sustain a faster and more adequate tissue regeneration, a positive feedback loop was described between the endothelial cells and satellite cells located near small blood vessels. Endothelial cells enable satellite cell proliferation through the secretion of growth factors, while differentiated myoblasts stimulate angiogenesis [85].

Lately, two studies, both conducted by injecting diphtheria toxin in mouse models, speculated that muscle repair is not possible without satellite cells, even under normal physiological conditions [142, 143]. During the experiments, neither non-satellite cells, nor the innervation and vasculature were altered. One of the studies developed mouse models in which only cells expressing Pax7 were killed by the toxin, while the second study crossed murine expressing an inducible diphtheria toxin with murine expressing under the control of Pax7 tamoxifen-inducible conditional recombinase [142, 143] . However, further studies are needed in order to undoubtably state that muscle restoration can only take place if satellite cells are present.

4.1 The regenerative muscle stem cell niche

In order to analyze the myogenic mechanism of the skeletal muscle, several injury models in mice were developed, including chemical injuries such as intramuscular injection of snake venoms notexin, cardiotoxin, and barium chloride, together with freeze injury and crash [144, 145]. The following regenerative response was found to comprise three phases: an inflammatory phase, a proliferative phase and, lastly, a differentiation phase.

Instantly after muscular damage, necrotic fibers hyper contract inside their basal lamina layer [146]. The remnant basal lamina is reconditioned by matrix remodeling enzymes and serves as a pattern for the development of new muscle fibers, and also guides the growth cones of motor neurons for reinnervation at original synaptic spots [147–153]. The necrosis of muscular fibers releases into circulation damage-associated molecular patters (DAMPs) that are tracked by both macrophages and mastocytes and mobilize neutrophils which deliver trophic factors to call up the satellite cells within 2 hours of damage [10, 154–156]. In this early phase of muscle regeneration, muscle tissue is cleansed of necrotic fibers through phagocytosis by macrophages and lymphocytes during this high inflammatory response phase [1, 147]. The proliferative stage is characterized by the expansion of stem cell niche and the generation of numerous transiently amplifying myoblasts which are waiting to differentiate [1]. The structural configuration of skeletal stem cell niche is modified by the accumulation of diverse components of the regenerative matrix. One of the components is represented by fibronectin, secreted by fibroblasts, satellite cells, and many other cells in the muscular tissue [157, 158]. Attachment to fibronectin is crucial for the prevention of anchorage-dependent cell's death, the regulation of asymmetric division and satellite cells segregation [159, 160]. Another component of the ECM is collagen VI secreted by fibroblasts, which is upregulated during the peak of satellite cells expansion and has essential mechanical properties in the skeletal muscle stem cell niche [161]. The satellite cells show a considerable proliferative ability in day 2 and 3 after an injury [10, 147]. Following the activation of satellite cells, monocytes convert into macrophages. M1 macrophages also exist in the mitogenic niche and secret VEGF, TNFα, IL-6, factors that are responsible for the limitation of early differentiation of myoblasts, stimulating the proliferation of stem cells instead [141, 162, 163]. When M2 macrophages become predominant to M1 macrophages, the first myoblasts start to differentiate [141, 164]. During the differentiation phase, myoblasts fuse to form multinucleated muscle cells and resident satellite cells and start to transit into a non-dividing state (quiescent state) [1]. At this point in the process of muscle regeneration, the blood vessels that irrigate the new muscle fibers become denser and well organized; smooth muscles and pericytes are initiated to sustain their structure, while immune cells limit the inflammatory reaction and secret anti-inflammatory cytokines to sustain tissue repair, resulting in the restoration of muscular architecture within nearly 2 weeks [10, 144, 147, 165–167].

4.2 Muscular stem cell niche in disease

The muscular stem cell niche suffers significant changes in muscle diseases such as inflammatory maladies, primary myopathies, and metabolic disorders [1]. The most notable, highly studied muscle pathologies are muscular dystrophies, defined by progressive muscle weakness caused by mutations in nuclear or sarcolemmal proteins such as dysferlin, dystrophin, and sarcoglycans, or by alterations of extracellular proteins [156]. Of these, the most common is Duchenne muscular dystrophy, an X-linked recessive disorder, diagnosed in early childhood, which is characterized by a progressive muscle-wasting process that affects skeletal muscles including diaphragm, limb, and heart muscles, in which death occurs in teenage years to 20s by cardiorespiratory failure [168]. In Duchenne disorder, the affected gene is dystrophin, which has an important structural function in anchoring the muscle fibers to the ECM in the muscular stem cell niche [13]. Moreover, dystrophin, which is expressed by satellite cells, is situated near the cell membrane and coordinates the flow of signaling molecules; therefore, a low level of dystrophin has a direct influence on the downstream cell-intrinsic signaling pathways of satellite cells, altering their functions [13, 169].

In most of the muscular dystrophies, the structural architecture of muscle cells is fragile, and fibers are doomed to get ruptured during repeated contractions; the stem cell niche is changing in such a way that the skeletal muscles get infiltrated with fat and fibrotic tissue [156, 170, 171]. Muscle ruptures are followed by protein leakage that activates inflammatory cells (lymphocytes, neutrophils, natural killer, macrophages) [172]. In muscular dystrophies, the inflammatory response is distinct than the one in trauma: there are many foci of injury developed in a continuous and asynchronous manner and the inflammatory process becomes chronic, and the ECM becomes thick and rigid, altering the muscular stem cell niche [173, 174]. In the extracellular environment, researchers discovered an accumulation of collagen I, III, IV, V, higher levels of various heparan sulfate proteoglycans and, moreover, a distinct regulation of the expression levels of MMPs and their endogenous inhibitor (TIMPs), together with various serine proteases and their endogenous inhibitors (serpins) [175–182]. Furthermore, the increased levels of matricellular proteins like fibrinogen, dermatopontin, asporin, and periostin were observed, together with a downregulation of fibrillin and nidogen [183–186]. The muscular stem cell niche is also enriched in signaling molecules during this inflammatory process, which influences the myoblast differentiation and fusion [155, 187]. For example, higher levels of prostaglandins, cytokines, and chemokines are described in muscular dystrophy, fact that supports the regenerative failure of dystrophic fibers [188–193]. This long-term inflammatory process changes the satellite cells in such manner that they can no longer compensate for the fiber degeneration, leading to an altered muscle functionality.

Diabetes mellitus represents a category of metabolic diseases characterized by a deficiency in insulin generation and function, leading to hyperglycemia, a condition which decreases the antioxidant level and increases the levels of free radical species [194, 195]. Muscle renewal is altered in type 1 and 2 of diabetes mellitus, these patients having a poor lesion-healing capacity [194, 196–198]. There is a fibrotic disposition of collagen and atypical levels of TNFα, TGFβ and ILs in diabetic or obese rats and patients due to the high level of M1 macrophages [199–202]. A sustained exposure to glucose generates an accumulation of glycated lipids and proteins that have an unfavorable impact on myoblasts from both rats and humans [203].

Another dramatic muscular pathology is cachexia. This state occurs as a consequence of various disorders such as AIDS, COPD, cancer, and heart failure and consists in the heavy and accelerated loss of striate muscle mass [204]. Muscular fibers from mice with neoplasms or from cachectic patients present abnormalities in the architecture of the basal lamina and in the membrane of the muscle cells, rather than infiltration of immune cells like in dystrophies or diabetes mellitus [205, 206]. This affected niche together with circulating plasma factors contributes to a hyperactivation of satellite cells and other non-satellite cells including pericytes. Furthermore, satellite cells constantly express Pax-7 self-renewal factor, an action that abolishes the differentiation process, leading to regenerative failure of muscular fibers [1].

Collectively, the data reviewed above showed the importance of stem cell niche behavior in the muscle regenerative process; yet further studies are required to fully understand these complex mechanisms involved in the renewal of normal and pathological muscle.

5. Perspectives

Over the last three decades, researchers found that satellite cells are a heterogenous population of stem cells and dedicated progenitors for myogenesis in striate muscle. With the development of new technologies, like single cell sequencing, mass cytometry, or super resolution imaging, the detailed study of satellite cells during growth, differentiation, and quiescence state is continuously improving [1]. The progress in discovering personalized therapies is slow and full of challenges, especially in the field of rare muscle pathologies, yet the stimulation of endogenous repair as a prospective therapy for muscle diseases should be one of the key perspectives that should be further looked into [207, 208]. The stem cell niche changes in behavior and composition during a lifetime, having tree periods: juvenile, adult, and old age. It is known that there are difficulties in muscular stem cells isolation and preservation due to the fact that they lose their myogenic ability after growing in vitro even for a short period of time [129]. A question that is yet to be answered is whether the use of juvenile stem cells instead of adult ones would provide for more adequate cell cultures, increasing plasticity and improving muscle regenerative therapies. For this purpose, and for a better understanding of skeletal stem cell niche, future challenging studies are needed.

6. Conclusion

The muscular stem cell niche is a remarkable structure that enables satellite cells and other non-satellite myogenic cells to repair and regenerate skeletal muscles when needed. As previously stated, the niche componence is highly variable, depending not only on the age of the body, but also on its well-being since a multitude of degenerative muscle disorders can alter the stem cell environment, leading to a decrease in the regenerative abilities of satellite cells. One of the elements of the niche that was proved to change during aging is the basal lamina, a key structure that apparently tends to interpose between the myofibers and satellite cells in older muscles, thus altering their communication, a fact that is believed to be associated to the latter's decrease in number. Furthermore, it was observed that in aged skeletal muscles, myofibers were decreased in mass, in contrast to the number of fibroblasts and adipocytes, which tended to increase. Satellite cells displayed diminished myogenic abilities and an accelerated apoptosis, probably due to lower expression levels of Pax7. Similar changes were described in degenerative muscle disorders, one of the most studied and severe being Duchenne muscular dystrophy. The chronic inflammation that appears in these diseases is believed to thicken the basal lamina and overflow the satellite cells with signaling molecules, impairing their capacity to restore muscle fibers. Other chronic disorders like diabetes mellitus and cachexia were also associated with niche alterations. Research in the field of regenerative medicine promises to innovate the therapies in these pathologies; however, there is a long way ahead and additional studies are needed.

Conflict of interest

The authors declare no conflict of interest.

Author details

Madalina-Gabriela Barbu[1,2†], Andreea-Elena Boboc[1†], Lidia Filip[1†], Oana-Larisa Bugnar[1], Dragos Cretoiu[1,3], Nicolae Suciu[1,4,5], Oana Daniela Toader[4,5], Sanda Maria Cretoiu[3*] and Silviu-Cristian Voinea[6]

1 Fetal Medicine Excellence Research Center, Alessandrescu-Rusescu National Institute for Mother and Child Health, Bucharest, Romania

2 Department of Rehabilitation Medicine, Ellias Emergency University Hospital, Bucharest, Romania

3 Department of Cell and Molecular Biology and Histology, Carol Davila University of Medicine and Pharmacy, Bucharest, Romania

4 Department of Obstetrics and Gynecology, Polizu Clinical Hospital, Alessandrescu-Rusescu National Institute for Mother and Child Health, Bucharest, Romania

5 Division of Obstetrics, Gynecology and Neonatology, Carol Davila University of Medicine and Pharmacy, Bucharest, Romania

6 Department of Surgical Oncology, Prof. Dr. Alexandru Trestioreanu Oncology Institute, Carol Davila University of Medicine and Pharmacy, Bucharest, Romania

*Address all correspondence to: sanda@cretoiu.ro

† Authors have contributed equally.

References

[1] Mashinchian O et al. The muscle stem cell niche in health and disease. Current Topics in Developmental Biology. 2018;**126**:23-65

[2] Yin H, Price F, Rudnicki MA. Satellite cells and the muscle stem cell niche. Physiological Reviews. 2013;**93**(1):23-67

[3] Schnyder S, Handschin C. Skeletal muscle as an endocrine organ: PGC-1alpha, myokines and exercise. Bone. 2015;**80**:115-125

[4] Betts JG, Peter D, Eddie J, Jody EJ, Oksana K, Dean HK et al. Chapter 10.2 Skeletal Muscle—Anatomy and Physiology. 2017. Available from: https://opentextbc.ca/anatomyandphysiology/chapter/10-2-skeletal-muscle/ [Cited: 14 July 2020]

[5] Rayagiri SS et al. Basal lamina remodeling at the skeletal muscle stem cell niche mediates stem cell self-renewal. Nature Communications. 2018;**9**(1):1075

[6] Moore KA, Lemischka IR. Stem cells and their niches. Science. 2006;**311**(5769):1880-1885

[7] Henze H et al. Skeletal muscle aging—Stem cells in the spotlight. Mechanisms of Ageing and Development. 2020;**189**:111283

[8] Mauro A. Satellite cell of skeletal muscle fibers. The Journal of Biophysical and Biochemical Cytology. 1961;**9**:493-495

[9] Abou-Khalil R et al. Role of muscle stem cells during skeletal regeneration. Stem Cells. 2015;**33**(5):1501-1511

[10] Shi X, Garry DJ. Muscle stem cells in development, regeneration, and disease. Genes & Development. 2006;**20**(13):1692-1708

[11] Buckingham M, Montarras D. Skeletal muscle stem cells. Current Opinion in Genetics & Development. 2008;**18**(4):330-336

[12] Dumont NA et al. Satellite cells and skeletal muscle regeneration. Comprehensive Physiology. 2015;**5**(3):1027-1059

[13] Almada AE, Wagers AJ. Molecular circuitry of stem cell fate in skeletal muscle regeneration, ageing and disease. Nature Reviews. Molecular Cell Biology. 2016;**17**(5):267-279

[14] Gopinath SD, Rando TA. Stem cell review series: Aging of the skeletal muscle stem cell niche. Aging Cell. 2008;**7**(4):590-598

[15] Yiu EM, Kornberg AJ. Duchenne muscular dystrophy. Journal of Paediatrics and Child Health. 2015;**51**(8):759-764

[16] Schofield R. The relationship between the spleen colony-forming cell and the haemopoietic stem cell. Blood Cells. 1978;**4**(1-2):7-25

[17] Papayannopoulou T, Scadden DT. Stem-cell ecology and stem cells in motion. Blood. 2008;**111**(8):3923-3930

[18] Holmberg J, Durbeej M. Laminin-211 in skeletal muscle function. Cell Adhesion & Migration. 2013;**7**(1):111-121

[19] Spradling A, Drummond-Barbosa D, Kai T. Stem cells find their niche. Nature. 2001;**414**(6859):98-104

[20] Scadden DT. The stem-cell niche as an entity of action. Nature. 2006;**441**(7097):1075-1079

[21] Yucel N, Blau HM. Chapter 18—Skeletal Muscle Stem Cells. In: Atala A et al., editors. Principles of Regenerative

Medicine. 3rd ed. Boston: Academic Press; 2019. pp. 273-293

[22] Samantha P, Marc F, Jeffrey G, Dale MR, Roger L, Michael T, et al. Practice Committee of the American Society for Reproductive Medicine. Endometriosis and Infertility: A Committee Opinion. Fertility and Sterility. 2012;**98**(3):591-598

[23] Endo T. Molecular mechanisms of skeletal muscle development, regeneration, and osteogenic conversion. Bone. 2015;**80**:2-13

[24] Buckingham M et al. The formation of skeletal muscle: From somite to limb. Journal of Anatomy. 2003;**202**(1):59-68

[25] Relaix F, Marcelle C. Muscle stem cells. Current Opinion in Cell Biology. 2009;**21**(6):748-753

[26] Relaix F et al. Divergent functions of murine Pax3 and Pax7 in limb muscle development. Genes & Development. 2004;**18**(9):1088-1105

[27] Kassar-Duchossoy L et al. Pax3/Pax7 mark a novel population of primitive myogenic cells during development. Genes & Development. 2005;**19**(12):1426-1431

[28] De Angelis L et al. Skeletal myogenic progenitors originating from embryonic dorsal aorta coexpress endothelial and myogenic markers and contribute to postnatal muscle growth and regeneration. The Journal of Cell Biology. 1999;**147**(4):869-878

[29] Ferrari G et al. Muscle regeneration by bone marrow-derived myogenic progenitors. Science. 1998;**279**(5356):1528-1530

[30] Grigoriadis AE, Heersche JN, Aubin JE. Differentiation of muscle, fat, cartilage, and bone from progenitor cells present in a bone-derived clonal cell population: Effect of dexamethasone. The Journal of Cell Biology. 1988;**106**(6):2139-2151

[31] Dellavalle A et al. Pericytes of human skeletal muscle are myogenic precursors distinct from satellite cells. Nature Cell Biology. 2007;**9**(3):255-267

[32] Berry SE et al. Multipotential mesoangioblast stem cell therapy in the mdx/utrn-/- mouse model for Duchenne muscular dystrophy. Regenerative Medicine. 2007;**2**(3):275-288

[33] Goodell MA et al. Isolation and functional properties of murine hematopoietic stem cells that are replicating in vivo. The Journal of Experimental Medicine. 1996;**183**(4):1797-1806

[34] Di Rocco G et al. Myogenic potential of adipose-tissue-derived cells. Journal of Cell Science. 2006;**119**(Pt 14): 2945-2952

[35] Otto A, Collins-Hooper H, Patel K. The origin, molecular regulation and therapeutic potential of myogenic stem cell populations. Journal of Anatomy. 2009;**215**(5):477-497

[36] Katz B. The terminations of the afferent nerve fibre in the muscle spindle of the frog. Philosophical Transactions of the Royal Society of London Series B, Biological Sciences. 1961;**243**(703):221-240

[37] Ishikawa H. Electron microscopic observations of satellite cells with special reference to the development of mammalian skeletal muscles. Zeitschrift für Anatomie und Entwicklungsgeschichte. 1966;**125**(1):43-63

[38] Moss FP, Leblond CP. Satellite cells as the source of nuclei in muscles of growing rats. The Anatomical Record. 1971;**170**(4):421-435

[39] Reznik M. Thymidine-3H uptake by satellite cells of regenerating skeletal muscle. The Journal of Cell Biology. 1969;**40**(2):568-571

[40] Konigsberg IR. Clonal analysis of myogenesis. Science. 1963;**140**(3573):1273-1284

[41] Snow MH. Myogenic cell formation in regenerating rat skeletal muscle injured by mincing. II. An autoradiographic study. The Anatomical Record. 1977;**188**(2):201-217

[42] Yaffe D. Cellular aspects of muscle differentiation in vitro. Current Topics in Developmental Biology. 1969;**4**:37-77

[43] Bischoff R. Regeneration of single skeletal muscle fibers in vitro. The Anatomical Record. 1975;**182**(2):215-235

[44] Konigsberg UR, Lipton BH, Konigsberg IR. The regenerative response of single mature muscle fibers isolated in vitro. Developmental Biology. 1975;**45**(2):260-275

[45] Jang YC et al. Skeletal muscle stem cells: Effects of aging and metabolism on muscle regenerative function. Cold Spring Harbor Symposia on Quantitative Biology. 2011;**76**:101-111

[46] Snow MH. Myogenic cell formation in regenerating rat skeletal muscle injured by mincing. I. A fine structural study. The Anatomical Record. 1977;**188**(2):181-199

[47] Darr KC, Schultz E. Exercise-induced satellite cell activation in growing and mature skeletal muscle. Journal of Applied Physiology (1985). 1987;**63**(5):1816-1821

[48] Rodgers JT et al. mTORC1 controls the adaptive transition of quiescent stem cells from G0 to GAlert. Nature. 2014;**510**(7505):393-396

[49] Alfaro LAS et al. CD34 promotes satellite cell motility and entry into proliferation to facilitate efficient skeletal muscle regeneration. Stem Cells. 2011;**29**(12):2030-2041

[50] McCune BK et al. Expression of transforming growth factor-beta isoforms in small round cell tumors of childhood. An immunohistochemical study. The American Journal of Pathology. 1993;**142**(1):49-58

[51] Mourkioti F, Rosenthal N. Rosenthal NIGF-1, inflammation and stem cells: Interactions during muscle regeneration. Trends in Immunology. 2005;**26**:535-542

[52] Chen SE, Jin B, Li YP. TNF-alpha regulates myogenesis and muscle regeneration by activating p38 MAPK. American Journal of Physiology. Cell Physiology. 2007;**292**(5):C1660-C1671

[53] Grounds M, Yablonka-Reuveni Z. Molecular and cell biology of muscle dystrophy. Molecular and Cell Biology of Human Diseases Series. 1993;**3**:210-256

[54] Fuchtbauer EM, Westphal H, Fuchtbauer EM, Westphal H. MyoD and myogenin are coexpressed in regenerating skeletal muscle of the mouse. Developmental Dynamics: An Official Publication of the American Association of Anatomists. 1992;**193**:34-39

[55] McCroskery S et al. Myostatin negatively regulates satellite cell activation and self-renewal. Journal of Cell Biology. 2003;**162**(6):1135-1147

[56] Buckingham M. Myogenic progenitor cells and skeletal myogenesis in vertebrates. Current Opinion in Genetics & Development. 2006;**16**(5):525-532

[57] Brack AS et al. A temporal switch from notch to Wnt signaling in muscle stem cells is necessary for normal

adult myogenesis. Cell Stem Cell. 2008;**2**(1):50-59

[58] Knudsen KA, Horwitz AF. Tandem events in myoblast fusion. Developmental Biology. 1977;**58**(2):328-338

[59] Lipton BH, Konigsberg IR. A fine-structural analysis of the fusion of myogenic cells. The Journal of Cell Biology. 1972;**53**(2):348-364

[60] Rash JE, Fambrough D. Ultra-structural and electrophysiological correlates of cell coupling and cytoplasmic fusion during myogenesis in vitro. Developmental Biology. 1973;**30**(1):166-186

[61] Schultz E. Satellite cell proliferative compartments in growing skeletal muscles. Developmental Biology. 1996;**175**(1):84-94

[62] Guasch G, Blanpain C. Defining the epithelial stem cell niche in skin. Medical Science (Paris). 2004;**20**(3):265-267

[63] Tajbakhsh S. Skeletal muscle stem and progenitor cells: Reconciling genetics and lineage. Experimental Cell Research. 2005;**306**(2):364-372

[64] Collins CA, Partridge TA. Self-renewal of the adult skeletal muscle satellite cell. Cell Cycle. 2005;**4**(10):1338-1341

[65] Halevy O et al. Pattern of Pax7 expression during myogenesis in the posthatch chicken establishes a model for satellite cell differentiation and renewal. Developmental Dynamics. 2004;**231**(3):489-502

[66] Olguin HC, Olwin BB. Pax-7 up-regulation inhibits myogenesis and cell cycle progression in satellite cells: A potential mechanism for self-renewal. Developmental Biology. 2004;**275**(2):375-388

[67] Zammit PS et al. Muscle satellite cells adopt divergent fates: A mechanism for self-renewal? The Journal of Cell Biology. 2004;**166**(3):347-357

[68] LaBarge MA, Blau HM. Biological progression from adult bone marrow to mononucleate muscle stem cell to multinucleate muscle fiber in response to injury. Cell. 2002;**111**(4):589-601

[69] Farrington-Rock C et al. Chondrogenic and adipogenic potential of microvascular pericytes. Circulation. 2004;**110**(15):2226-2232

[70] Doherty MJ et al. Vascular pericytes express osteogenic potential in vitro and in vivo. Journal of Bone and Mineral Research. 1998;**13**(5):828-838

[71] Kutcher ME, Herman IM. The pericyte: Cellular regulator of microvascular blood flow. Microvascular Research. 2009;**77**(3):235-246

[72] Díaz-Manera J et al. The increase of pericyte population in human neuromuscular disorders supports their role in muscle regeneration in vivo. The Journal of Pathology. 2012;**228**(4):544-553

[73] Kohfeldt E et al. Nidogen-2: A new basement membrane protein with diverse binding properties. Edited by Holland IB. Journal of Molecular Biology. 1998;**282**(1):99-109

[74] Ghadiali RS et al. Dynamic changes in heparan sulfate during muscle differentiation and ageing regulate myoblast cell fate and FGF2 signalling. Matrix Biology. 2017;**59**:54-68

[75] Blanco-Bose WE et al. Purification of mouse primary myoblasts based on α7 integrin expression. Experimental Cell Research. 2001;**265**(2):212-220

[76] Carey DJ. Syndecans: Multifunctional cell-surface co-receptors. Biochemical Journal. 1997;**327**(1):1-16

[77] Xian X, Gopal S, Couchman JR. Syndecans as receptors and organizers of the extracellular matrix. Cell and Tissue Research. 2009;**339**(1):31

[78] Nunes AM et al. Impaired fetal muscle development and JAK-STAT activation mark disease onset and progression in a mouse model for merosin-deficient congenital muscular dystrophy. Human Molecular Genetics. 2017;**26**(11):2018-2033

[79] Rooney JE et al. Severe muscular dystrophy in mice that lack dystrophin and α7 integrin. Journal of Cell Science. 2006;**119**(11):2185-2195

[80] Shefer G, Wleklinski-Lee M, Yablonka-Reuveni Z. Skeletal muscle satellite cells can spontaneously enter, an alternative mesenchymal pathway. Journal of Cell Science. 2004;**117**:5393-5404

[81] Pisani DF et al. The topoisomerase 1-interacting protein BTBD1 is essential for muscle cell differentiation. Cell Death & Differentiation. 2004;**11**(11):1157-1165

[82] Brack AS et al. Increased Wnt signaling during aging alters muscle stem cell fate and increases fibrosis. Science. 2007;**317**(5839):807-810

[83] Goldspink G et al. Age-related changes in collagen gene expression in the muscles of mdx dystrophic and normal mice. Neuromuscular Disorders. 1994;**4**(3):183-191

[84] Greco AV et al. Insulin resistance in morbid obesity: Reversal with intramyocellular fat depletion. Diabetes. 2002;**51**(1):144-151

[85] Christov C et al. Muscle satellite cells and endothelial cells: Close neighbors and privileged partners. Molecular Biology of the Cell. 2007;**18**(4):1397-1409

[86] Chazaud B et al. Satellite cells attract monocytes and use macrophages as a support to escape apoptosis and enhance muscle growth. The Journal of Cell Biology. 2003;**163**(5):1133-1143

[87] Germani A et al. Vascular endothelial growth factor modulates skeletal myoblast function. The American Journal of Pathology. 2003;**163**(4):1417-1428

[88] Takahashi A et al. Myogenic Akt signaling regulates blood vessel recruitment during myofiber growth. Molecular and Cellular Biology. 2002;**22**(13):4803-4814

[89] Borisov AB, Dedkov EI, Carlson BM. Interrelations of myogenic response, progressive atrophy of muscle fibers, and cell death in denervated skeletal muscle. The Anatomical Record. 2001;**264**(2):203-218

[90] Carlson BM et al. Skeletal muscle regeneration in very old rats. The Journals of Gerontology. Series A, Biological Sciences and Medical Sciences. 2001;**56**(5):B224-B233

[91] Sonnet C et al. Human macrophages rescue myoblasts and myotubes from apoptosis through a set of adhesion molecular systems. Journal of Cell Science. 2006;**119**(Pt 12):2497-2507

[92] Darmani H et al. Expression of nitric oxide synthase and transforming growth factor-beta in crush-injured tendon and synovium. Mediators of Inflammation. 2004;**13**(5-6):299-305

[93] Sinha-Hikim I et al. Effects of testosterone supplementation on skeletal muscle fiber hypertrophy and satellite cells in community-dwelling older men. The Journal of Clinical Endocrinology and Metabolism. 2006;**91**(8):3024-3033

[94] Jones DL, Wagers AJ. No place like home: Anatomy and function of

the stem cell niche. Nature Reviews. Molecular Cell Biology. 2008;**9**(1):11-21

[95] Snow MH. The effects of aging on satellite cells in skeletal muscles of mice and rats. Cell and Tissue Research. 1977;**185**(3):399-408

[96] Conboy IM et al. Notch-mediated restoration of regenerative potential to aged muscle. Science. 2003;**302**(5650):1575-1577

[97] Taylor-Jones JM et al. Activation of an adipogenic program in adult myoblasts with age. Mechanisms of Ageing and Development. 2002;**123**(6):649-661

[98] Jejurikar SS et al. Aging increases the susceptibility of skeletal muscle derived satellite cells to apoptosis. Experimental Gerontology. 2006;**41**(9):828-836

[99] Robert L, Labat-Robert J. Aging of connective tissues: From genetic to epigenetic mechanisms. Biogerontology. 2000;**1**(2):123-131

[100] Schultz MB, Sinclair DA. When stem cells grow old: Phenotypes and mechanisms of stem cell aging. Development (Cambridge, England). 2016;**143**(1):3-14

[101] Tajbakhsh S, Cossu G. Establishing myogenic identity during somitogenesis. Current Opinion in Genetics & Development. 1997;**7**(5):634-641

[102] Musumeci G et al. Somitogenesis: From somite to skeletal muscle. Acta Histochemica. 2015;**117**(4-5):313-328

[103] Chargé SB, Rudnicki MA. Cellular and molecular regulation of muscle regeneration. Physiological Reviews. 2004;**84**(1):209-238

[104] Katz B. The termination of the afferent nerve fibre in the muscle spindle of the frog. Philosophical Transactions of the Royal Society of London Series B, Biological Sciences. 1961;**243**(703):221-240

[105] Forcina L et al. An overview about the biology of skeletal muscle satellite cells. Current Genomics. 2019;**20**(1):24-37

[106] Seale P et al. Pax7 is required for the specification of myogenic satellite cells. Cell. 2000;**102**(6):777-786

[107] Relaix F et al. Pax3 and Pax7 have distinct and overlapping functions in adult muscle progenitor cells. The Journal of Cell Biology. 2006;**172**(1):91-102

[108] Irintchev A et al. Expression pattern of M-cadherin in normal, denervated, and regenerating mouse muscles. Developmental Dynamics. 1994;**199**(4):326-337

[109] Garry DJ et al. Persistent expression of MNF identifies myogenic stem cells in postnatal muscles. Developmental Biology. 1997;**188**(2):280-294

[110] Mechtersheimer G, Staudter M, Möller P. Expression of the natural killer cell-associated antigens CD56 and CD57 in human neural and striated muscle cells and in their tumors. Cancer Research. 1991;**51**(4):1300-1307

[111] Tatsumi R et al. HGF/SF is present in normal adult skeletal muscle and is capable of activating satellite cells. Developmental Biology. 1998;**194**(1):114-128

[112] Jesse TL et al. Interferon regulatory factor-2 is a transcriptional activator in muscle where it regulates expression of vascular cell adhesion molecule-1. The Journal of Cell Biology. 1998;**140**(5):1265-1276

[113] Beauchamp JR et al. Expression of CD34 and Myf5 defines the majority of quiescent adult skeletal muscle satellite cells. The Journal of Cell Biology. 2000;**151**(6):1221-1234

[114] Cornelison DD et al. Syndecan-3 and syndecan-4 specifically mark skeletal muscle satellite cells and are implicated in satellite cell maintenance and muscle regeneration. Developmental Biology. 2001;**239**(1):79-94

[115] Schmidt K et al. Sox8 is a specific marker for muscle satellite cells and inhibits myogenesis. The Journal of Biological Chemistry. 2003;**278**(32):29769-29775

[116] Lee HJ et al. Sox15 is required for skeletal muscle regeneration. Molecular and Cellular Biology. 2004;**24**(19):8428-8436

[117] Sherwood RI et al. Isolation of adult mouse myogenic progenitors: Functional heterogeneity of cells within and engrafting skeletal muscle. Cell. 2004;**119**(4):543-554

[118] Volonte D, Liu Y, Galbiati F. The modulation of caveolin-1 expression controls satellite cell activation during muscle repair. The FASEB Journal. 2005;**19**(2):237-239

[119] Fukada S et al. Molecular signature of quiescent satellite cells in adult skeletal muscle. Stem Cells. 2007;**25**(10):2448-2459

[120] Gnocchi VF et al. Further characterisation of the molecular signature of quiescent and activated mouse muscle satellite cells. PLoS One. 2009;**4**(4):e5205

[121] Fukada S et al. Hesr1 and Hesr3 are essential to generate undifferentiated quiescent satellite cells and to maintain satellite cell numbers. Development. 2011;**138**(21):4609-4619

[122] Dumont NA et al. Dystrophin expression in muscle stem cells regulates their polarity and asymmetric division. Nature Medicine. 2015;**21**(12):1455-1463

[123] Bischoff R, Heintz C. Enhancement of skeletal muscle regeneration. Development Dynamics. 1994;**201**(1): 41-54

[124] Bischoff R. Interaction between satellite cells and skeletal muscle fibers. Development. 1990;**109**(4):943-952

[125] Collins CA et al. A population of myogenic stem cells that survives skeletal muscle aging. Stem Cells. 2007;**25**(4):885-894

[126] Rochlin K, Yu S, Roy S, Baylies MK. Developmental Biology. 2010;**341**:66-83

[127] Wang YX, Rudnicki MA. Nature Reviews. Molecular Cell Biology. 2011;**13**:127-133

[128] Cooper ST, McNeil PL. Physiological Reviews. 2015;**95**:1205-1240

[129] Montarras D et al. Direct isolation of satellite cells for skeletal muscle regeneration. Science. 2005;**309**:2064-2067

[130] Relaix F et al. A Pax3/Pax7-dependent population of skeletal muscle progenitor cells. Nature. 2005;**435**:948-953

[131] Gayraud-Morel B et al. A role for the myogenic determination gene Myf5 in adult regenerative myogenesis. Developmental Biology. 2007;**312**:13-28

[132] Ustanina S, Carvajal J, Rigby P, Braun T. The myogenic factor Myf5 supports efficient skeletal muscle regeneration by enabling transient myoblast amplification. Stem Cells. 2007;**25**:2006-2016

[133] Sacco A, Doyonnas R, Kraft P, Vitorovic S, Blau HM. Self-renewal and expansion of single transplanted muscle stem cells. Nature. 2008;**456**:502-506. A report demonstrating that a single satellite cell is sufficient to restore a functional satellite cell pool

[134] Collins CA et al. Stem cell function, self-renewal, and behavioral heterogeneity of cells from the adult muscle satellite cell niche. Cell. 2005;**122**:289-301

[135] Gussoni E et al. Dystrophin expression in the mdx mouse restored by stem cell transplantation. Nature. 1999;**401**:390-394

[136] Benchaouir R et al. Restoration of human dystrophin following transplantation of exon-skipping-engineered DMD patient stem cells into dystrophic mice. Cell Stem Cell. 2007;**1**:646-657

[137] Sampaolesi M et al. Cell therapy of alpha-sarcoglycan null dystrophic mice through intra-arterial delivery of mesoangioblasts. Science. 2003;**301**:487-492

[138] Sampaolesi M et al. Mesoangioblast stem cells ameliorate muscle function in dystrophic dogs. Nature. 2006;**444**:574-579

[139] Torrente Y. Human circulating AC133+ stem cells restore dystrophin expression and ameliorate function in dystrophic skeletal muscle. Journal of Clinical Investigation. 2004;**114**:182-195

[140] Dellavalle A et al. Pericytes resident in postnatal skeletal muscle differentiate into muscle fibres and generate satellite cells. Nature Communications. 2011;**2**:499

[141] Arnold L et al. Inflammatory monocytes recruited after skeletal muscle injury switch into antiinflammatory macrophages to support myogenesis. The Journal of Experimental Medicine. 2007;**204**:1057-1069

[142] Sambasivan R et al. Pax7-expressing satellite cells are indispensable for adult skeletal muscle regeneration. Development. 2011;**138**:3647-3656

[143] Lepper C et al. An absolute requirement for Pax7-positive satellite cells in acute injury-induced skeletal muscle regeneration. Development. 2011;**138**:3639-3646

[144] Hardy D, Besnard A, Latil M, Jouvion G, Briand D, Thepenier C, et al. Comparative study of injury models for studying muscle regeneration in mice. PLoS One. 2016;**11**:e0147198

[145] Lukjanenko L, Brachat S, Pierrel E, Lach-Trifilieff E, Feige JN. Genomic profiling reveals that transient adipogenic activation is a hallmark of mouse models of skeletal muscle regeneration. PLoS One. 2013;**8**:e71084

[146] Bischoff R. Interaction between satellite cells and skeletal muscle fibers. Development. 1990;**109**:943-952

[147] Goetsch SC, Hawke TJ, Gallardo TD, Richardson JA, Garry DJ. Transcriptional profiling and regulation of the extracellular matrix during muscle regeneration. Physiological Genomics. 2003;**14**:261-271

[148] Kherif S, Lafuma C, Dehaupas M, Lachkar S, Fournier JG, Verdiere-Sahuque M, et al. Expression of Matrix Metalloproteinases 2 and 9 in Regenerating Skeletal Muscle: A Study in Experimentally Injured and mdxMuscles. Developmental Biology. 1999;**205**:158-170

[149] Caldwell CJ, Mattey DL, Weller RO. Role of the basement membrane in the regeneration of skeletal muscle. Neuropathology and Applied Neurobiology. 1990;**16**:225-238

[150] Koskinen SO, Ahtikoski AM, Komulainen J, Hesselink MK, Drost MR, Takala TE. Short-term effects of forced eccentric contractions on collagen synthesis and degradation in rat skeletal muscle. Pflügers Archiv: European Journal of Physiology. 2002;**444**:59-72

[151] Sanes JR, Marshall LM, McMahan UJ. Reinnervation of muscle fiber basal lamina after removal of myofibers. Differentiation of regenerating axons at original synaptic sites. The Journal of Cell Biology. 1978;**78**:176-198

[152] Vracko R, Benditt EP. Basal lamina: The scaffold for orderly cell replacement: Observations on regeneration of injured skeletal muscle fibers and capillaries. The Journal of Cell Biology. 1972;**55**:406-419

[153] Webster MT, Manor U, Lippincott-Schwartz J, Fan CM. Intravital imaging reveals ghost fibers as architectural units guiding myogenic progenitors during regeneration. Cell Stem Cell. 2016;**18**:243-252

[154] Tidball JG, Dorshkind K, Wehling-Henricks M. Shared signaling systems in myeloid cell-mediated muscle regeneration. Development. 2014;**141**:1184-1196

[155] Tidball JG, Villalta SA. Regulatory interactions between muscle and the immune system during muscle regeneration. American journal of physiology. Regulatory, Integrative and Comparative Physiology. 2010;**298**:R1173-R1187

[156] Pannérec A, Marazzi G, Sassoon D. Stem cells in the hood: The skeletal muscle niche. Trends in Molecular Medicine. 2012;**18**:599-606. DOI: 10.1016/j.molmed.2012.07.004

[157] Lukjanenko L, Jung MJ, Hegde N, Perruisseau-Carrier C, Migliavacca E, Rozo M, et al. Loss of fibronectin from the aged stem cell niche affects the regenerative capacity of skeletal muscle in mice. Nature Medicine. 2016;**22**:897-905

[158] Singh P, Carraher C, Schwarzbauer JE. Assembly of fibronectin extracellular matrix. Annual Review of Cell and Developmental Biology. 2010;**26**:397-419

[159] Bentzinger CF, Wang YX, von Maltzahn J, Soleimani VD, Yin H, Rudnicki MA. Fibronectin regulates Wnt7a signaling and satellite cell expansion. Cell Stem Cell. 2013;**12**:75-87

[160] Yennek S, Burute M, Thery M, Tajbakhsh S. Cell adhesion geometry regulates non-random DNA segregation and asymmetric cell fates in mouse skeletal muscle stem cells. Cell Reports. 2014;**7**:961-970

[161] Urciuolo A, Quarta M, Morbidoni V, Gattazzo F, Molon S, Grumati P, et al. Collagen VI regulates satellite cell self-renewal and muscle regeneration. Nature Communications. 2013;**4**:1964

[162] Chazaud B, Sonnet C, Lafuste P, Bassez G, Rimaniol AC, Poron F, et al. Satellite cells attract monocytes and use macrophages as a support to escape apoptosis and enhance muscle growth. The Journal of Cell Biology. 2003;**163**:1133-1143

[163] Saclier M, Yacoub-Youssef H, Mackey AL, Arnold L, Ardjoune H, Magnan M, et al. Differentially activated macrophages orchestrate myogenic precursor cell fate during human skeletal muscle regeneration. Stem Cells. 2013;**31**:384-396

[164] Tidball JG. Nature reviews. Immunology. 2007;**17**:165-178

[165] Luque E, Pena J, Martin P, Jimena I, Vaamonde R. Capillary supply during development of individual regenerating muscle fibers. Anatomia, Histologia, Embryologia. 1995;**24**:87-89

[166] Birbrair A, Zhang T, Wang ZM, Messi ML, Mintz A, Delbono O. Pericytes: multitasking cells in the regeneration of injured, diseased, and

aged skeletal muscle. Frontiers in Aging Neuroscience. 2014;**6**:245

[167] Deng B, Wehling-Henricks M, Villalta SA, Wang Y, Tidball JG. IL-10 triggers changes in macrophage phenotype that promote muscle growth and regeneration. Journal of Immunology. 2012;**189**:3669-3680

[168] Watkins SC, Cullen MJ. A quantitative study of myonuclear and satellite cell nuclear size in Duchenne's muscular dystrophy, polymyositis and normal human skeletal muscle. The Anatomical Record. 1988;**222**:6-11

[169] Sacco A et al. Short telomeres and stem cell exhaustion model Duchenne muscular dystrophy in mdx/mTR mice. Cell. 2010;**143**:1059-1071. A report introducing the dystrophin/Tert1-deficient mouse as a better model that more closely recapitulates the human disorder DMD, and providing evidence that stem cell depletion exacerbates DMD symptoms

[170] Sahenk Z, Mendell JR. The muscular dystrophies: Distinct pathogenic mechanisms invite novel therapeutic approaches. Current Rheumatology Reports. 2011;**13**:199-207

[171] Rahimov F, Kunkel LM. The cell biology of disease: Cellular and molecular mechanisms underlying muscular dystrophy. The Journal of Cell Biology. 2013;**201**:499-510

[172] Tidball JG. Inflammatory processes in muscle injury and repair. American Journal of Physiology-Regulatory, Integrative and Comparative Physiology. 2005;**288**:R345-R353

[173] Serrano AL, Munoz-Canoves P. Fibrosis development in early-onset muscular dystrophies: Mechanisms and translational implications. Seminars in Cell & Developmental Biology. 2017;**64**:181-190

[174] Dadgar S, Wang Z, Johnston H, Kesari A, Nagaraju K, Chen YW, et al. Asynchronous remodeling is a driver of failed regeneration in Duchenne muscular dystrophy. The Journal of Cell Biology. 2014;**207**:139-158

[175] Peltonen L, Myllyla R, Tolonen U, Myllyla VV. Changes in collagen metabolism in diseased muscle: II. Immunohistochemical studies. Archives of Neurology. 1982;**39**:756-759

[176] Myllyla R, Myllyla VV, Tolonen U, Kivirikko KI. Changes in collagen metabolism in diseased muscle: I. Biochemical studies. Archives of Neurology. 1982;**39**:752-755

[177] Alvarez K, Fadic R, Brandan E. Augmented synthesis and differential localization of heparan sulfate proteoglycans in Duchenne muscular dystrophy. Journal of Cellular Biochemistry. 2002;**85**:703-713

[178] Caceres S, Cuellar C, Casar JC, Garrido J, Schaefer L, Kresse H, et al. Synthesis of proteoglycans is augmented in dystrophic mdx mouse skeletal muscle. European Journal of Cell Biology. 2000;**79**:173-181

[179] Alameddine HS, Morgan JE. Matrix metalloproteinases and tissue inhibitor of metalloproteinases in inflammation and fibrosis of skeletal muscles. Journal of Neuromuscular Diseases. 2016;**3**:455-473

[180] Fukushima K, Nakamura A, Ueda H, Yuasa K, Yoshida K, Takeda S, et al. Activation and localization of matrix metalloproteinase-2 and-9 in the skeletal muscle of the muscular dystrophy dog (CXMD J). BMC Musculoskeletal Disorders. 2007;**8**:54

[181] Sun GL, Zhao S, Li P, Jiang HK. Expression of tissue inhibitor of metalloproteinase-1 in progression

muscular dystrophy. Neuroscience Bulletin. 2006;**22**:85-90

[182] von Moers A, Zwirner A, Reinhold A, Bruckmann O, van Landeghem F, Stoltenburg-Didinger G, et al. Increased mRNA expression of tissue inhibitors of metalloproteinase-1 and-2 in Duchenne muscular dystrophy. Acta Neuropathologica. 2005;**109**:285-293

[183] Holland A, Murphy S, Dowling P, Ohlendieck K. Pathoproteomic profiling of the skeletal muscle matrisome in dystrophinopathy associated myofibrosis. Proteomics. 2016;**16**:345-366

[184] Holland A, Dowling P, Meleady P, Henry M, Zweyer M, Mundegar RR, et al. Proteomics. Label-free mass spectrometric analysis of the mdx-4cv diaphragm identifies the matricellular protein periostin as a potential factor involved in dystrophinopathy-related fibrosis. 2015;**15**:2318-2331

[185] Thakur R, Mishra DP. Matrix reloaded: CCN, tenascin and SIBLING group of matricellular proteins in orchestrating cancer hallmark capabilities. Pharmacology & Therapeutics. 2016;**168**:61-74

[186] Arecco N, Clarke CJ, Jones FK, Simpson DM, Mason D, Beynon RJ, et al. Elastase levels and activity are increased in dystrophic muscle and impair myoblast cell survival, proliferation and differentiation. Scientific Reports. 2016;**6**:24708

[187] Villalta SA, Rosenberg AS, Bluestone JA. The immune system in Duchenne muscular dystrophy: Friend or foe. Rare Diseases. 2015;**3**:e1010966

[188] McArdle A, Foxley A, Edwards RH, Jackson MJ. Prostaglandin metabolism in dystrophin-deficient MDX mouse muscle. Biochemical Society Transactions. 1991;**19**:177S

[189] Nakagawa T, Takeuchi A, Kakiuchi R, Lee T, Yagi M, Awano H, et al. A prostaglandin D2 metabolite is elevated in the urine of Duchenne muscular dystrophy patients and increases further from 8 years old. Clinica Chimica Acta. 2013;**423**:10-14

[190] Okinaga T, Mohri I, Fujimura H, Imai K, Ono J, Urade Y, et al. Induction of hematopoietic prostaglandin D synthase in hyalinated necrotic muscle fibers: Its implication in grouped necrosis. Acta Neuropathologica. 2002;**104**:377-384

[191] Kuru S, Inukai A, Kato T, Liang Y, Kimura S, Sobue G. Expression of tumor necrosis factor-α in regenerating muscle fibers in inflammatory and non-inflammatory myopathies. Acta Neuropathologica. 2003;**105**:217-224

[192] Kumar A, Boriek AM. Mechanical stress activates the nuclear factor-kappa B pathway in skeletal muscle fibers: A possible role in Duchenne muscular dystrophy. The FASEB Journal. 2003;**17**:386-396

[193] Villalta SA, Rinaldi C, Deng B, Liu G, Fedor B, Tidball JG. Interleukin-10 reduces the pathology of mdx muscular dystrophy by deactivating M1 macrophages and modulating macrophage phenotype. Human Molecular Genetics. 2011;**20**:790-805

[194] Aragno M, Mastrocola R, Catalano MG, Brignardello E, Danni O, Boccuzzi G. Oxidative stress impairs skeletal muscle repair in diabetic rats. Diabetes. 2004;**53**:1082-1088

[195] Henriksen EJ, Diamond-Stanic MK, Marchionne EM. Oxidative stress and the etiology of insulin resistance and type 2 diabetes. Free Radical Biology & Medicine. 2011;**51**:993-999

[196] Jeong J, Conboy MJ, Conboy IM. Pharmacological inhibition of myostatin/TGF-β receptor/pSmad3 signaling rescues muscle regenerative responses in mouse model of type 1 diabetes. Acta Pharmacologica Sinica. 2013;**34**:1052-1060

[197] Krause MP, Al-Sajee D, D'Souza DM, Rebalka IA, Moradi J, Riddell MC, et al. Impaired macrophage and satellite cell infiltration occurs in a muscle-specific fashion following injury in diabetic skeletal muscle. PLoS One. 2013;**8**:e70971

[198] Nunan R, Harding KG, Martin P. Clinical challenges of chronic wounds: Searching for an optimal animal model to recapitulate their complexity. Disease Models & Mechanisms. 2014;**7**:1205-1213

[199] Berria R, Wang L, Richardson DK, Finlayson J, Belfort R, Pratipanawatr T, et al. Increased collagen content in insulin-resistant skeletal muscle. American journal of physiology. Endocrinology and Metabolism. 2006;**290**:E560-E565

[200] Hong EG, Ko HJ, Cho YR, Kim HJ, Ma Z, Yu TY, et al. Interleukin-10 prevents diet-induced insulin resistance by attenuating macrophage and cytokine response in skeletal muscle. Diabetes. 2009;**58**:2525-2535

[201] Richardson DK, Kashyap S, Bajaj M, Cusi K, Mandarino SJ, Finlayson J, et al. Lipid infusion decreases the expression of nuclear encoded mitochondrial genes and increases the expression of extracellular matrix genes in human skeletal muscle. The Journal of Biological Chemistry. 2005;**280**:10290-10297

[202] Watts R, McAinch AJ, Dixon JB, O'Brien PE, Cameron-Smith D. Increased Smad signaling and reduced MRF expression in skeletal muscle from obese subjects. Obesity (Silver Spring). 2013;**21**:525-528

[203] Chiu CY, Yang RS, Sheu ML, Chan DC, Yang TH, Tsai KS, et al. Advanced glycation end-products induce skeletal muscle atrophy and dysfunction in diabetic mice via a RAGE-mediated, AMPK-down-regulated, Akt pathway. The Journal of Pathology. 2016;**238**:470-482

[204] Morley JE, Thomas DR, Wilson MM. Cachexia: Pathophysiology and clinical relevance. The American Journal of Clinical Nutrition. 2006;**83**:735-743

[205] Acharyya S, Butchbach ME, Sahenk Z, Wang H, Saji M, Carathers M, et al. Dystrophin glycoprotein complex dysfunction: A regulatory link between muscular dystrophy and cancer cachexia. Cancer Cell. 2005;**8**:421-432

[206] He WA, Berardi E, Cardillo VM, Acharyya S, Aulino P, Thomas-Ahner J, et al. NF-κB–mediated Pax7 dysregulation in the muscle microenvironment promotes cancer cachexia. The Journal of Clinical Investigation. 2013;**123**:4821-4835

[207] Niks EH, Aartsma-Rus A. Exon skipping: A first in class strategy for Duchenne muscular dystrophy. Expert Opinion on Biological Therapy. 2017;**17**: 225-236

[208] Bello L, Pegoraro E. Genetic diagnosis as a tool for personalized treatment of Duchenne muscular dystrophy. Acta Myologica. 2016;**35**:122-127

Chapter 3

Sarcopenia in Older Adults

Eli Carmeli

Abstract

Sarcopenia has become of great interest and focus of many studies since this phenomenon affects many people. Moreover, sarcopenia is associated with two more pandemic phenomena: frailty and obesity. These health-related conditions are increasing in western countries in general and in the older population in particular. Each of such health conditions relates to functional decline, yet the combination of two or three of them in one person severely affects quality of life and longevity. Aged individuals who are less physically active are more likely to develop sarcopenic obesity, and those who are obese with muscle weakness and inactive are disposed to become frail individuals. Hence, frailty and obesity overlap profoundly with the physical manifestations of sarcopenia of aging. These "unhappy" triads encompasses a wider range of geriatric decline that also includes cognitive, psychology and social deterioration associated with adverse outcomes. Nevertheless, this chapter focuses only on sarcopenia and will review the pathophysiological background of age-related decline in muscle mass and strength.

Keywords: sarcopenia, elderly, strength, muscle mass, physical performance, radicals, cytokines

1. Introduction

1.1 The "unhappy triad"

The end of the last century and the beginning of the first two decades of the present century were characterized by the rise of three medical or health pandemic phenomena, each of which has a serious impact on public health and especially among older people. These three conditions are frailty, sarcopenia, and obesity. When sarcopenia or frailty is also accompanied by obesity, a sarcopenic/frail-obese phenotype is established [1]. Moreover, the presence of these "unhappy triads" of health conditions, in one person, poses a significant threat to one's quality of life and longevity. The prevalence of each of such conditions (i.e., frailty, sarcopenia, and obesity) is widely estimated within different countries; however, with no one single best outcome measure for these diagnoses, there is highly wide range of manifestation and diagnoses in each of these health phenomena [2].

A "cycle of sarcopenia" may be created in which in the presence of one or two factors such as frailty and or obesity, sarcopenia status is likely to continue to deteriorate unless there is outside intervention. It is extremely difficult to overcome this "unhappy triad" when the affected people do not have the resources necessary to get out of muscle weakness and fatigue, such as lower cardiac function (myocardial infraction, angina, chronic heart failure, metabolic state (hypertension, diabetes, and obesity) and arthritis.

IntechOpen

Longevity steadily increased over the past several decades. Life expectancy in 65 year Western country subjects is ~20 years, and the proportion of people over age 60 is increasing faster than any other groups (2). Obesity is also worldwide growing [3] and is also accompanied by significant alterations in body composition, with a decline in lean body mass and muscle strength and with an increase in fat mass. This phenomenon known as sarcopenic obesity [4].

The concept of frailty syndrome is basically a geriatric syndrome, which is recently becoming one of the dominant concepts in advanced age. Frailty is a dynamic condition with the presence of several components. There are two major operational definitions for frailty. The most widely used concept is the Fried physical frailty phenotype, which defines frailty based on three or more of the following five symptoms: unintentional weight loss, slowness, weakness, exhaustion, and low physical activity [5]. Yet, functional decline due to sarcopenia is in the core of frailty syndrome [6].

This chapter focuses on sarcopenia. Aged skeletal muscles can be induced to die through different mechanisms mainly via two systems, apoptosis or autophagy; both systems can be activated through different molecules such as free radicals, inflammatory molecules, hormones, and others [7].

2. Sarcopenia

There are currently over 10,000 articles published in referee journals dealing with the phenomenon of Sarcopenia, which was first proposed by Irwin Harold Rosenberg in 1989 at the annual conference of the American Society for Clinical Nutrition. Sarcopenia is age-related myopenia (decrease of muscle mass) and dynapenia (decrease in muscle strength) [8]. More specifically, sarcopenia is a health problem of old people characterized by a slow, progressive skeletal muscle disorder involving the accelerated loss of muscle mass and strength followed by the functional decline that is associated with falls, obesity, frailty, frequent hospitalization, and mortality [9]. Sarcopenia has become of great interest and focus of many studies and since this phenomenon affects many people, the number of older population with sarcopenia is expected to increase all over the world, and it is becoming one of the important and interests, and causes a great deal of financial burden, a private and a public concern, from the individual level to the state and various institutions that deal with welfare and health [10]. It predisposed by genetic profile and lifestyle factors occurring across the life course [11]. The expression of Let-7b and Let-7e microRNA precursors (regulating muscle apoptosis) is significantly higher in older versus younger subjects. Ingenuity pathway analysis identified that the Let-7 family predicted gene targets were related to pathways and biological functions associated with macrophages activity.

Therefore, a great deal of knowledge about the nature of the phenomenon was accumulated, from a biological and clinical point of view, different means to diagnose it, and with particular ways to treat it such as nutritional interventions and drugs to augment the beneficial effects of resistance exercise.

2.1 Definition of sarcopenia

Sarcopenia (Greek "sarx" or flesh + "penia" or loss) is a geriatric syndrome which is described as a progressive decline in skeletal muscle mass and muscle strength from approximately the fifth decade of life.

The European Working Group on Sarcopenia in Older People (EWGSOP) defined sarcopenia in 2010 as a quote: "a syndrome characterized by progressive and generalized loss of skeletal muscle mass and strength with the risk of adverse outcome such as physical disability, poor quality of life, and death" [12]. The EWGSOP proposed that age-related muscle weakness is considered as "primary sarcopenia" when no other reason is evident except aging itself. EWGSOP also suggests a concept of three phases of sarcopenia: pre-sarcopenia (there is low muscle mass without low muscle strength or decline in physical performance); sarcopenia (low muscle mass, accompanying either low muscle strength or low physical performance); and severe sarcopenia (when all three criteria are detected).

Another consensus definition of primary sarcopenia done by the International Working Group for Sarcopenia (IWGS) as "an individual presents functional and mobility decline, history of recurrent falls, recent unwanted body weight loss, recent-hospitalization, and chronic metabolic diseases (e.g., diabetes, hypothyroid) malnutrition, low protein intake, and cancer" [13].

2.2 Prevalence and epidemiology of sarcopenia

It is well known and extensively documented that as an older person reaches his sixth decade of life, there is a progressive decline in muscle mass (~1% per year) and strength (~2.5–3% per year) [14]. Sarcopenia is more prevalent in men than in women. It is more prevalent in large muscle groups such as tight, more in untrained individuals and more in people with poor health background [15]. There is a strong association between, muscle strength, age, gender, and disability. In general, there is a decrease in muscle mass at an annual rate of 1.5% after about 50 years old, reaching to 3% per year in their eight decade [16].

Public health planners, physicians and researchers are needed to come up with the consensus of criteria for estimating the prevalence of sarcopenia. Moreover, at present time, there are lacking data for developing any consensus on what constitutes poor muscle mass, and what is the optimal, valid, and reliable tool to measure and to diagnose sarcopenia.

The prevalence of sarcopenia needs to be investigated in multiethnic population, and to explore association with obesity, socioeconomic status, mental and cognitive function, morbidity, quality of life, and life style. Previous studies have been demonstrated associations between muscle mass and function, whereas other studies have established associations between the following:

a. sarcopenia and physical activity [17],

b. muscle mass and BMI [18];

c. muscle performance and certain minerals [19];

d. muscle mass and strength and depressive symptoms and [20];

e. sarcopenia and cognitive impairment [21];

f. muscle strength and falls [22];

g. muscle mass and osteoporosis [23], thus those with sarcopenia possessed approximately 13 times higher risk of having osteoporosis [24], and there is a significant association between osteoporosis and deterioration of the skeletal microarchitecture [25]. The prevalence of osteosarcopenia increases with aged men and women [26]; and

h. sarcopenia and meat intake in male and milk intake in female [27].

3. Biological mechanisms of sarcopenia: from molecular to histological level

There are several molecular mechanisms that may be involved, in some degree, in the commencement and development of sarcopenia. Although the molecular and cellular mechanisms underlying sarcopenia still remain to be clarified, certain common biological mechanisms have been suggested to be involved in sarcopenia. This section will include, in brief, the most common mechanisms related to sarcopenia: oxidative stress [reactive oxygen and nitrogen species (ROS and RNS)]; a-without clinical symptoms of muscle fiber inflammation (due to presence of myokines/cytokines like TNF-α and IL-6); hormonal regulation impairment (such as testosterone, growth hormone, IGF-1, glutathione 4, insulin resistance, and vitamin D); vitamin E deficiency; proteolysis pathway [the lack of responsiveness of the ubiquitin-proteasome system and alterations in the regulation of autophagy and apoptotic pathway (Bcl2 signaling and NF-*K*b)]; and finally, the role of adult stem (satellite) cells. Identifying these mechanisms and their underlying origins is expected to facilitate strategy of intervention programs [28].

From a physiology and histology point of view, the skeletal muscle comprises several types of fibers. The most prominent types are type I and type II fibers. Type II fast twitch muscle fibers characterized by high glycolytic potential, lower oxidative capacity, and faster response, are aimed at muscle strength and short-duration anaerobic activities, whereas type I slow twitch muscle fibers are known as fatigue-resistant due to their characteristics such as large density of capillary bed and myoglobin and being abundant with mitochondria, to better supply oxygen and nutrients to the muscle, thus to improve muscular endurance and aerobic activities [29].

Sarcopenia is characterized by more hypotrophy and less fiber activation of the lower extremity muscles than upper limbs. Moreover, the lower limb muscles of old people are smaller and have significantly more fats and connective tissues than lower limb muscles in young individuals. Sarcopenia is characterized by a reduction in both the number and size of muscle fibers, mainly of type II, and is to some extent caused by a slowly progressive myogenic process, which is stem cells dependent. Therefore, these changes affect not only in energy production, poor muscle repair, and deprived fiber regeneration, but also practically in decline in physical performance and in functional capacity such as walking (stairs), running, and early onset of fatigue which all associate with poor quality of life and more dependency [30].

Of course there is a connection and interdependence between the various factors. Sometimes one of them is a cause or effect, and sometimes it is a result of or outcome from. Some of the mechanisms have a positive correlation and others have a negative correlation. In general, skeletal muscle can "die" in different molecular pathways. Sarcopenia, as a normal physiological process, is associated with a significant rise in the levels of inflammatory molecules both in blood serum and intra- and extracellular. The aging process induced oxidative stress (OS) and degradation of damaged mitochondria promotes the accumulation of lipofuscin, which is one histological marker of fiber oxidative damage. The accumulation of lipofuscin, is recognized as the hallmark pigment of aging muscle. Lipofuscin is an intralysosomal, composed of cross-linked protein residues and lipid per oxidized molecules. This intracellular waste material interferes with muscle metabolism and muscle contraction [31].

Oxidative stress resulted due to imbalance between the production of reactive oxygen/nitrogen species and antioxidants/nitrogen defense molecules. Consequently and practically, a chain response of inflammatory molecules appears within the fibers with the release of myokines such as tumor necrosis factor-α (TNF-α), interleukin-6 (IL-6), and interleukin-1 (IL-1) that lead to a predisposition to age-related sarcopenia afterward through the activation of the ubiquitin-protease system and the activation of myofiber signaling pathway that leads to muscle apoptosis. It is also suggested that cytokines also contributes to anabolic resistance through provoking the anabolic effect mediated by insulin growth factor-1 (IGF-1), involving in growth hormone resistance which limits IGF-I availability. Some other potential factors and mechanisms are suggested leading to sarcopenia such as TGF-β-activated kinase (TAK)-1; C-reactive protein; a significant reduction of dihydropyridine (DHP)-sensitive Ca^{2+} (the decrease of Ca^{2+} available for mechanical responses in aged skeletal muscle is due to DHP receptor (DHPR)-ryanodine receptor (RyR) uncoupling); and the stress of sarcoplasmic reticulum due to accumulation of unfolded or misfolded proteins like heat shock proteins.

3.1 Oxidative stress and sarcopenia

Sarcopenia is a multifactorial event, thus redox signaling and oxidative stress have a key role play, due to an increase in reactive oxygen and nitrogen species (ROS/RNS) levels, a decrease in enzymatic antioxidant protection and followed by myofiber "quiet" inflammation (i.e., the presence of myokines). Therefore, the oxidative stress is more extensively described in the below section of this chapter.

3.1.1 Endogenous sources of reactive oxygen species, reactive nitrogen species, and antioxidant systems

Reactive oxygen species (ROS) are mainly and normally produced by the mitochondria, and a normal ROS level is indispensable for myofiber functions.

The mitochondrial electron transport chain transfer of a single electron to molecular oxygen gives rise to a monovalent reduction of oxygen, which leads to the formation of superoxide ions (O_2.−). It is the first step in the chain of events to create more free radicals such as hydrogen peroxide (H_2O_2), hydroxyl radical (OH.), and hydroxyl ion (OH^-) [32]. Another source of ROS in skeletal muscle is a large NOX family enzymes (NOX_1, NOX_2, and NOX_4) located in the sarcoplasmic reticulum, transverse tubule, and also in the sarcoplasma membrane [33]. These enzymes have the capacity to transport electrons across the sarcoplasma membrane and generate superoxide and other downstream reactive oxygen species (ROS). Since these enzymes play an important role in excitation contraction coupling, hyperexpression or overproduction of NOXs inhibits muscle contractions. Another mechanism that can explain the crosstalk between NOXs and ROS production is the rise of intracellular Ca^{2+} levels by NOX-derived ROS, which, increasing mitochondrial Ca^{2+} load, induces the ROS production by these organelles.

Reactive nitrogen species (RNS) derived from nitric oxide (•NO) and superoxide ions is produced via the enzymatic activity of inducible nitric oxide synthase 2 (NOS_2) and nicotinamide adenine dinucleotide phosphate oxidase (NADPH oxidase) [34]. NOS_2 is also expressed after induction of cytokines [26]. In skeletal muscle, there are three different isoforms of this isoenzyme: endothelial NOS (eNOS), neuronal NOS (nNOS), and inducible isoform (iNOS). RNS arise from several sources and the levels increase with contractile activity. Nitric oxide (NO) is formed from L-arginine in a reaction catalyzed by the nitric oxide synthase (NOS) enzyme, and it is an important cell signaling molecule [35].

The intrinsic and extrinsic antioxidant systems inhibit oxidation [36, 37]. The intrinsic system includes enzymes such as superoxide dismutase, catalase, peroxidase, and glutathione. Manganese superoxide dismutase (MnSOD) is synthesized by a mitochondrion that catalyzes the breakdown of the superoxide anion into oxygen and hydrogen peroxide. Catalase catalyzes the conversion of hydrogen peroxide to water and oxygen, peroxidase catalyzes the reduction of hydrogen peroxide, and glutathione is a very efficient scavenger of hydrogen peroxide, while glutathione peroxidase 4 is most active with lipid hydroperoxides. The extrinsic system includes dietary supplements such as Ubiquinone-10, coenzyme Q10, creatine, and others, and the combination with physical exercise is even better for muscle atrophy prevention and/or treatment of sarcopenia [38].

The levels of ROS and RNS inside the fibers are firmly controlled by the balance between the rate of endogenous synthesis by ROS/RNS generating systems and the rate of removal through the nonenzymatic and enzymatic antioxidant systems [39]. In aged muscles, there is an excessive ROS/RNS production or diminishing of antioxidant production which interrupts the myofiber metabolism and physiological function, both in resting and in force production [40]. There is plenty of evidence that sarcopenia is caused by an increase of endogenous ROS and/or RNS formation, on the one hand, and decrease in quantity, quality, and antioxidant system efficiency, on the other hand [41, 42]. Sarcopenia is also characterized by mitochondrial dysfunction; mitochondrial morphological changes, lacking fusion and fission; less mitochondria mobility, leading to the accumulation of damaged mitochondria that induces a catabolic process; muscle loss; and fiber inflammation [43, 44].

In conclusion, age-related ROS and RNS overproduction not only generates damage of muscle but also plays a role in regulating intracellular signal transduction pathways that are directly or indirectly involved in skeletal muscle inflammation and apoptosis.

3.1.2 The role of cytokines in sarcopenia

Sarcopenia is definitely associated with inflammatory cytokines/myokines, which prompt a serious negative consequence as a loss of muscle mass and strength with concomitant increase in fat mass, eventually stimulating protein catabolism and muscle degeneration. As such, an excepted catabolic inflammatory process is often observed in older adults, and it can enhance and deteriorate the status of sarcopenia [45].

Skeletal muscle tissue is an vital source of inflammatory molecules, known as "myokines" (e.g., IL-6, IL-1b, TNFα, and IL-1ra) which are overexpressed in aged skeletal muscles, related to the slow, non symptomatic, slowly progressed, inflammation process demonstrated in elderly individuals. Myokines are secreted in response to muscle contraction or strength training [46]; however, their activation as inflammatory signal pathways happen due to aging, which reveals their critical impact on sarcopenia [47]. Several inflammatory myokines, especially interleukin-1 6, and 10 (IL-1, Il-6, IL-10), tumor necrosis factor-alpha (TNF-α), and myostatin play crucial roles in the modulation of inflammatory signaling pathway during the aging-related loss of skeletal muscle [48, 49].

3.1.2.1 Interleukin

The relationship between sarcopenia and the inflammatory cytokines interleukin-1 and 6 (IL-1, IL-6), and the anti-inflammatory cytokine interleukin-10 (IL-10) in an elderly population is well reported [50, 51]. IL-6 within the muscle fibers promotes glucose uptake and fat oxidation via the phosphoinositide 3-kinase (PI3K) and AMP-activated protein kinase (AMPK) signaling pathways, respectively, and improves insulin sensitivity by blocking the proinflammatory signaling pathways in the muscle. High levels of IL-6 (>40 pg./ml) and IL-10 (>4 pg./ml) are associated with lower physical performance, muscle strength, and muscle mass [52]. Hospitalized geriatric patients with inflammation represented significantly weaker muscle function, shoulder extension strength, and a worse fatigue resistance [53]. Old people living in nursing homes and long-term-assisted living facilities presenting high IL-6 levels were associated with the higher prevalence of frailty [54]. The significant role of IL-6 levels on depressive symptoms in older women in the year after hip fracture may represent a sickness syndrome that is chronic in some individuals [55]. A recent study in community-dwelling older men suggested that the high levels of interleukin-1 (IL-1) is associated with a low grip strength [56]. The ratio of proinflammatory cytokine IL-6 to anti-inflammatory cytokine IL-10 (IL-6/IL-10 ratio) >9.5 pg./ml has been used as a reliable marker for measuring inflammatory status [57].

IL-10 is an anti-inflammatory myokine, mostly produced by macrophages, T-helper 2 cells (also known as CD4+ cells), B-lymphocytes, and monocytes. These cells either secrete antibodies or suppress and destroy any immune response. IL-10 is responsible for destroying the proinflammatory response in various tissues, including skeletal muscle, by suppressing the activation of phagocytes such as macrophages and releasing and activating the inflammatory cytokines such as IL-6, TNFα, and IL-1β. Increased IL-10 was associated with poor physical performance [58, 59].

In summary, inflammatory and proinflammatory interleukin cytokines have both been linked with a number of age-related outcomes, including sarcopenia, chronic morbidity, functional decline, and mortality [60].

3.1.2.2 Tumor necrosis factor-α (TNF α)

The appearance of sarcopenia is accompanied by the increased levels of inflammation factors such as TNF-α. TNF-α inhibits the synthesis of muscle proteins, accelerates protein decomposition, and upregulates the expression of muscle growth inhibitory factor myostatin and muscle atrophy proteins, F-box-1 Atrogin-1, etc., so as to accelerate protein catabolism and promote skeletal muscle consumption. TNF-α and its soluble receptors showed the most consistent associations with decline in muscle mass and strength [61]. TNF-α is also reported to suppress the Akt/mTOR pathway [62], promoting muscle catabolism, oxidative stress, and nitric acid production [63].

3.1.2.3 C-reactive protein (CRP)

Elevated levels of these proteins, reflecting the conditions of chronic inflammation, have been associated with reduced muscle mass and strength [64], decreased physiology capacity, and more difficulties in performing the activities of daily living [65]. The levels of CRP are negatively associated with appendicular lean body mass [66]. In addition, the increased levels of lipid peroxidation result in the breakdown of biological phospholipids in sarcolemma and mitochondrial membrane, thus preventing the mitochondria to break down and converting fatty acid molecules (β-oxidation) to acyl-CoA chains in order to produce energy. Damage to mitochondria also increases the formation of reactive oxygen species such as superoxide anion [$O_2{\cdot}-$], hydroxyl radical [OH−]), and hydrogen peroxide [H_2O_2], complemented by the increased production and secretion of proinflammatory cytokines such as tissue necrosis factor (TNF)-α and IL-1, 6, and 8 that trigger a cytokine cascade of the inflammatory cytokines that worsen the insulin resistance in skeletal muscle, resulting in the decrease of aerobic capacity [67].

3.2 Hormones and sarcopenia

A variety of other hormones appear to play roles in the age-related alterations in muscle mass, strength function, and in the regulation of muscle metabolism [68].

Testosterone appears to be the central hormone involved in the development of sarcopenia. Testosterone is an important physiologic steroid hormone in muscle mass maintenance. Endogenous testosterone which naturally produced within the endocrine system in both men and women decline gradually with age, correlating with decreased muscle strength it increases both muscle mass and activates adult stem cells (i.e., satellite cells) leading to improved muscle function [69].

Normal growth hormone (GH) level is associated with notable protection from age-related disease in general, and more specifically against sarcopenia. The levels of GH and GH binding proteins declines upon aging. Growth hormone deficiency leads to the loss of muscle mass but not muscle strength [69, 70].

Skeletal muscle is the major organ in which the insulin-mediated glucose uptake by glucose transporter 4 (GLUT4) takes place. Lack of insulin, or IGF-1, or insulin resistance leads to accelerated development of sarcopenia. The muscle IGF-I level declines in aged population.

The primary action of insulin in skeletal muscle is to stimulate glucose uptake and metabolism. In physiological condition as insulin resistance, there is a gradual muscle wasting by several mechanisms such as the following: (a) suppression of PI3K/Akt signaling leading to the activation of caspase-3 and the ubiquitin-proteasome proteolytic pathway causing muscle protein degradation; (b) beta-adrenergic stimulation increases the lipolysis of the cell membrane, breaking down G-proteins that lead to interfering with growth hormone/insulin growth factor-1 receptor bind and diminished muscle regeneration; (c) advancement of gluconeogenesis metabolic pathway; (d) upregulation of sterol regulatory element-binding protein 1c (SREBP-1c); and (e) altering triglyceride and cholesteryl esters transport in the core of plasma lipoproteins, which causes triglycerides to accumulate in skeletal muscle [71, 72]. It has been reported that IGF-I drops 1.88 ng/ml/year in men and 2.13 ng/ml/year in women [73]. Circulating IGF-I level was found to be significantly reduced in sarcopenia patients [74]. mTOR signaling is a significant factor in sarcopenia, and mTOR signaling is altered by the change of IGF-I level [75].

Various medical problems and health conditions such as muscle weakness reduced the muscle mass that is predominantly a type II muscle fiber, bone pain, and systematic oxidative stress linked to 1,25-dihydroxyvitamin D [1,25(OH)2D]/vitamin D deficiency. The vitamin D deficiency expands the sarcomeres space that allows the infiltration of irregular connective tissue and fat tissue. As such, the vitamin D deficiency resulting in reducing physical performance such as gait speed and cognitive performance (such as sustained attention and speed of information processing), mental well-being (e.g., depression), falls and leading to bone deformities. The vitamin D deficiency is a serious medical condition that drastically affects the quality of life of older adults. There are a number of reasons that play a role in vitamin D deficiencies in older adults. Since the majority of the time they spend indoors, they get minimal exposure to sunlight, lacking resistance exercise which is well known to preserve muscle function, and their skin is less exposed to the synthesis of vitamin D [76, 77].

3.3 Vitamin E

Vitamin E, which is a group of eight fat soluble compounds, four tocopherols (α, β, γ, and δ) and four tocotrienols (α, β, γ, and δ), is a lipid soluble vitamin, with potent antioxidant properties and has a role in the modulation of signaling pathways. The vitamin E molecules deficiency, due to malabsorption or malnutrition, worsens age-associated skeletal dysfunction and enhances muscle degeneration, thus increasing sarcopenia [78, 79].

4. Conclusions

This chapter reviewed the possible mechanisms that are linked to sarcopenia. The etiology of sarcopenia is multifactorial, including a wide range of both intramuscular and extra muscular factors. This chapter focuses only on the intramuscular factors that include oxidative stress, inflammation, lack of vitamins, and hormones. Extra muscular factors include adult stem cells, extra cellular matrix (e.g., the function of matrix metaloproteinases), capillary bed, and neuronal activity.

Conflict of interest

The author declares no conflicts of interest, financial or otherwise.

Author details

Eli Carmeli
Department of Physical Therapy, University of Haifa, Israel

*Address all correspondence to: ecarmeli@univ.haifa.ac.il

References

[1] Buch A, Keinan-Boker L, Kis O, Carmeli E, Izkhakov E, Ish-Shalom M, et al. Severe central obesity or diabetes can replace weight loss in the detection of frailty in obese younger elderly - a preliminary study. Clinical Interventions in Aging. 2018;**13**:1907-1918

[2] Buch A, Carmeli E, Shefer G, Keinan-Boker L, Berner Y, Marcus Y, et al. Cognitive impairment and the association between frailty and functional deficits are linked to abdominal obesity in the elderly. Maturitas. 2018;**114**:46-53

[3] Pizzol D, Smith L, Fontana L, Caruso MG, et al. Associations between body mass index, waist circumference and erectile dysfunction: A systematic review and META-analysis. Reviews in Endocrine & Metabolic Disorders. 2020;**31**. [Epub ahead of print]

[4] Batsis JA, Villareal DT. Sarcopenic obesity in older adults: Aetiology, epidemiology and treatment strategies. Nature Reviews. Endocrinology. 2018;**14**(9):513-537

[5] Fried LP, Tangen CM, Walston J, Newman AB, et al. Frailty in older adults: Evidence for a phenotype. The Journals of Gerontology. Series A, Biological Sciences and Medical Sciences. 2001;**56**(3):M146-M157

[6] Michel JP, Ecarnot F. Integrating functional ageing into daily clinical practice. Journal of Frailty, Sarcopenia and Falls. 2019;**4**(2):30-35

[7] Carmeli E, Aizenbud D, Rom O. How do skeletal muscles die? An overview. Advances in Experimental Medicine and Biology. 2015;**861**:99-111

[8] Rosenberg IH. Diagnosis, treatment, and prevention of sarcopenia. The American Journal of Clinical Nutrition. 1989;**50**(5):1231-1233

[9] Papadopoulou SK. Sarcopenia: A contemporary health problem among older adult populations. Nutrients. 2020;**12**(5). pii: E1293

[10] Beaudart C, Zaaria M, Pasleau F, Reginster JY, Bruyère O. Health outcomes of sarcopenia: A systematic review and meta-analysis. PLoS One. 2017;**12**(1):e0169548

[11] Drummond MJ, McCarthy JJ, Sinha M, Spratt HM, Volpi E, Esser KA, et al. Aging and microRNA expression in human skeletal muscle: A microarray and bioinformatics analysis. Physiological Genomics. 2011;**43**(10):595-603

[12] Cruz-Jentoft AJ, Baeyens JP, Bauer JM, Boirie Y, et al. Sarcopenia: European consensus on definition and diagnosis: Report of the European working group on sarcopenia in older people. Age and Ageing. 2010;**39**:412-423

[13] Fielding RA, Vellas B, Evans WJ, Bhasin S, et al. Sarcopenia: An undiagnosed condition in older adults. Current consensus definition: Prevalence, etiology, and consequences. International Working Group on Sarcopenia. Journal of the American Medical Directors Association. 2011;**12**:249-256

[14] Daly RM, Rosengren BE, Alwis G, Ahlborg HG, Sernbo I, Karlsson MK. Gender specific age-related changes in bone density, muscle strength and functional performance in the elderly: A-10 year prospective population-based study. BMC Geriatrics. 2013;**13**:71

[15] Ligthart-Melis GC, Luiking YC, Kakourou A, Cederholm T, Maier AB, de van der Schueren MAE. Frailty,

sarcopenia, and malnutrition frequently (co-)occur in hospitalized older adults: A systematic review and meta-analysis. Journal of the American Medical Directors Association. 2020; pii: S1525-8610(20)30251-30256

[16] Sehl ME, Yates FE. Rates of senescence between ages 30 and 70 years in healthy people. The Journals of Gerontology. Series A, Biological Sciences and Medical Sciences. 2001;**56**:198-208

[17] Steffl M, Bohannon RW, Sontakova L, Tufano JJ, Shiells K, Holmerova I. Relationship between sarcopenia and physical activity in older people: A systematic review and meta-analysis. Clinical Interventions in Aging. 2017;**12**:835-845

[18] Iannuzzi-Sucich M, Prestwood KM, Kenny AM. Prevalence of sarcopenia and predictors of skeletal muscle mass in healthy, older men and women. The Journals of Gerontology. Series A, Biological Sciences and Medical Sciences. 2002;**57**(12):M772-M777

[19] van Dronkelaar C, van Velzen A, Abdelrazek M, et al. And physical performance in older adults: A systematic review. Journal of the American Medical Directors Association. 2018;**19**(1):6-11.e3

[20] Taani MH, Siglinsky E, Kovach CR, Buehring B. Psychosocial factors associated with reduced muscle mass, strength, and function in residential care apartment complex residents. Research in Gerontological Nursing. 2018;**11**(5):238-248

[21] Chang KV, Hsu TH, Wu WT, Huang KC, Han DS. Association between sarcopenia and cognitive impairment: A systematic review and meta-analysis. Journal of the American Medical Directors Association. 2016;**17**(12):1164.e7-1164.e15

[22] Zhang XM, Cheng ASK, Dou Q, Zhang W, Zeng Y. "Sarcopenia and its association with falls and fractures in older adults: A systematic review and meta-analysis" by Yeung et al. Journal of Cachexia, Sarcopenia and Muscle. 2020;**11**(1):330-331

[23] Nielsen BR, Abdulla J, Andersen HE, Schwarz P, Suetta C. Sarcopenia and osteoporosis in older people: A systematic review and meta-analysis. European Geriatric Medicine. 2018;**9**:419-434

[24] Sjöblom S, Suuronen J, Rikkonen T, Honkanen R, Kröger H, Sirola J. Relationship between postmenopausal osteoporosis and the components of clinical sarcopenia. Maturitas. 2013;**75**:175-180

[25] Locquet M, Beaudart C, Reginster J-Y, Bruyère O. Association between the decline in muscle health and the decline in bone health in older individuals from the SarcoPhAge cohort. Calcified Tissue International. 2019;**104**:273-284

[26] Kirk B, Al Saedi A, Duque G. Osteosarcopenia: A case of geroscience. Aging Medicine (Milton). 2019;**2**(3):147-156

[27] Lim HS. Association of dietary variety status and sarcopenia in Korean elderly. Journal of Bone Metabolism. 2020;**27**(2):143-149

[28] Riuzzi F, Sorci G, Arcuri C, Giambanco I, Bellezza I, Minelli A, et al. Cellular and molecular mechanisms of sarcopenia: The S100B perspective. Journal of Cachexia, Sarcopenia and Muscle. 2018;**9**(7):1255-1268

[29] Carter CS, Justice JN, Thompson L. Lipotoxicity, aging, and muscle contractility: Does fiber type matter? Geroscience. 2019;**41**(3):297-308

[30] Lexell J. Human aging, muscle mass, and fiber type composition.

The Journals of Gerontology. Series A, Biological Sciences and Medical Sciences. 1995;**50**:11-16

[31] Hütter E, Skovbro M, Lener B, Prats C, Rabøl R, Dela F, et al. Oxidative stress and mitochondrial impairment can be separated from lipofuscin accumulation in aged human skeletal muscle. Aging Cell. 2007;**6**(2):245-256

[32] Sakellariou GK, McDonagh B. Redox homeostasis in age-related muscle atrophy. Advances in Experimental Medicine and Biology. 2018;**1088**:281-306

[33] Sullivan-Gunn MJ, Lewandowski PA. Elevated hydrogen peroxide and decreased catalase and glutathione peroxidase protection are associated with aging sarcopenia. BMC Geriatrics. 2013;**13**:104

[34] Nemes R, Koltai E, Taylor AW, Suzuki K, Gyori F, Radak Z. Reactive oxygen and nitrogen species regulate key metabolic, anabolic, and catabolic pathways in skeletal muscle. Antioxidants (Basel). 2018;**7**(7). pii: E85

[35] Hall DT, Ma JF, Marco SD, Gallouzi IE. Inducible nitric oxide synthase (iNOS) in muscle wasting syndrome, sarcopenia, and cachexia. Aging (Albany NY). 2011;**3**(8):702-715

[36] Fougere B, van Kan GA, Vellas B, Cesari M. Redox systems, antioxidants and sarcopenia. Current Protein & Peptide Science. 2018;**19**(7):643-648

[37] Di Meo S, Napolitano G, Venditti P. Physiological and pathological role of ROS: Benefits and limitations of antioxidant treatment. International Journal of Molecular Sciences. 2019;**20**(19). pii: E4810

[38] Guescini M, Tiano L, Genova ML, Polidori E, Silvestri S, Orlando P, et al. The combination of physical exercise with muscle-directed antioxidants to counteract sarcopenia: A biomedical rationale for pleiotropic treatment with creatine and coenzyme Q10. Oxidative Medicine and Cellular Longevity. 2017;**2017**:7083049

[39] Ji LL. Antioxidant signaling in skeletal muscle: A brief review. Experimental Gerontology. 2007;**42**(7):582-593

[40] Ji LL. Modulation of skeletal muscle antioxidant defense by exercise: Role of redox signaling. Free Radical Biology & Medicine. 2008;**44**(2):142-152

[41] Liguori I, Russo G, Curcio F, Bulli G, Aran L, Della-Morte D, et al. Oxidative stress, aging, and diseases. Clinical Interventions in Aging. 2018;**13**:757-772

[42] Belenguer-Varea Á, Tarazona-Santabalbina FJ, Avellana-Zaragoza JA, Martínez-Reig M, Mas-Bargues C, Inglés M. Oxidative stress and exceptional human longevity: Systematic review. Free Radical Biology & Medicine. 2020;**149**:51-63

[43] Azuma K, Ikeda K, Inoue S. Functional mechanisms of mitochondrial respiratory chain supercomplex assembly factors and their involvement in muscle quality. International Journal of Molecular Sciences. 2020;**21**(9). pii: E3182

[44] Abrigo J, Simon F, Cabrera D, Vilos C, Cabello-Verrugio C. Mitochondrial dysfunction in skeletal muscle pathologies. Current Protein & Peptide Science. 2019;**20**(6):536-546

[45] Beenakker KG, Ling CH, Meskers CG, de Craen AJ, Stijnen T, Westendorp RG, et al. Patterns of muscle strength loss with age in the general population and patients with a chronic inflammatory state. Ageing Research Reviews. 2010;**9**(4):431-436

[46] Raschke S, Eckardt K, Bjorklund Holven K, Jensen J, Eckel J. Identification and validation of novel contraction-regulated myokines released from primary human skeletal muscle cells. PLoS One. 2013;**8**(4):e62008

[47] Beyer I, Mets T, Bautmans I. Chronic low-grade inflammation and age-related sarcopenia. Current Opinion in Clinical Nutrition and Metabolic Care. 2012;**15**:12-22

[48] Lee JH, Jun HS. Role of myokines in regulating skeletal muscle mass and function. Frontiers in Physiology. 2019;**10**:42

[49] Coelho-Junior HJ, Picca A, Calvani R, Uchida MC, Marzetti. If my muscle could talk: Myokines as a biomarker of frailty. Experimental Gerontology. 2019;**127**:110715

[50] Lambernd S, Taube A, Schober A, Platzbecker B, Gorgens SW, Schlich R, et al. Contractile activity of human skeletal muscle cells prevents insulin resistance by inhibiting pro-inflammatory signalling pathways. Diabetologia. 2012;**55**:1128-1139

[51] Rong YD, Bian AL, Hu HY, Ma Y, Zhou XZ. Study on relationship between elderly sarcopenia and inflammatory cytokine IL-6, anti-inflammatory cytokine IL-10. BMC Geriatrics. 2018;**18**(1):308

[52] Raj DS, Dominic EA, Pai A, Osman F, Morgan M, et al. Muscle, cytokines, and oxidative stress in end-stage renal disease. Kidney International. 2005;**68**(5):2338-2344

[53] Lustosa LP, Batista PP, Pereira DS, Pereira LSM, Scianni A, Ribeiro-Samora GA. Comparison between parameters of muscle performance and inflammatory biomarkers of non-sarcopenic and sarcopenic elderly women. Clinical Interventions in Aging. 2017;**12**:1183-1191

[54] Bautmans I, Njemini R, Lambert M, Demanet C, Mets T. Circulating acute phase mediators and skeletal muscle performance in hospitalized geriatric patients. The Journals of Gerontology. Series A, Biological Sciences and Medical Sciences. 2005;**60**(3):361-367

[55] Langmann GA, Perera S, Ferchak MA, Nace DA, Resnick NM, Greenspan SL. Inflammatory markers and frailty in long-term care residents. Journal of the American Geriatrics Society. 2017;**65**(8):1777-1783

[56] Matheny ME, Miller RR, Shardell MD, Hawkes WG, Lenze EJ, Magaziner J, et al. Inflammatory cytokine levels and depressive symptoms in older women in the year after hip fracture: Findings from the Baltimore hip studies. Journal of the American Geriatrics Society. 2011;**59**(12):2249-2255

[57] Patel HP, Al-Shanti N, Davies LC, Barton SJ, Grounds MD, Tellam RL, et al. Lean mass, muscle strength and gene expression in community dwelling older men: Findings from the Hertfordshire sarcopenia study (HSS). Calcified Tissue International. 2014;**95**(4):308-316

[58] Sun J, Su J, Xie Y, Yin MT, Huang Y, Xu L, et al. Plasma IL-6/IL-10 ratio and IL-8 LDH, and HBDH level predict the severity and the risk of death in AIDS patients with pneumocystis pneumonia. Journal of Immunology Research. 2016;**2016**:1583951

[59] Dong B, Sun B. Inflammatory markers and disability in Chinese older adults. Journal of Gerontology & Geriatric Research. 2016;**5**:275

[60] Wilson D, Jackson T, Sapey E, Lord JM. Frailty and sarcopenia: The

potential role of an aged immune system. Ageing Research Reviews. 2017;**36**:1-10

[61] Rong YD, Bian AL, Hu HY, Ma Y, Zhou XZ. Study on relationship between elderly sarcopenia and inflammatory cytokine IL-6, anti-inflammatory cytokine IL-10. BMC Geriatrics. 2018;**18**:308

[62] Schaap LA, Pluijm SM, Deeg DJ, Harris TB, et al. Health ABC study. The Journals of Gerontology. Series A, Biological Sciences and Medical Sciences. 2009;**64A**(11):1183-1189

[63] Ziaaldini MM, Marzetti E, Picca A, Murlasits Z. Biochemical pathways of sarcopenia and their modulation by physical exercise: A narrative review. Frontiers in Medicine (Lausanne). 2017;**4**:167

[64] Hall DT, Ma JF, Marco SD, Gallouzi IE. Inducible nitric oxide synthase (iNOS) in muscle wasting syndrome, sarcopenia, and cachexia. Aging (Albany NY). 2011;**3**(8):702-715

[65] Schaap LA, Pluijm SM, Deeg DJ, Visser M. Inflammatory markers and loss of muscle mass (sarcopenia) and strength. The American Journal of Medicine. 2006;**119**(6):526.e9-17

[66] Cesari M, Penninx BW, Pahor M, Lauretani F, Corsi AM, Rhys Williams G, et al. Inflammatory markers and physical performance in older persons: The in CHIANTI study. The Journals of Gerontology. Series A, Biological Sciences and Medical Sciences. 2004;**59**(3):242-248

[67] Bano G, Trevisan C, Carraro S, Solmi M, Luchini C, Stubbs B, et al. Maturitas. 2017;**96**:10-15

[68] Kob R, Bollheimer LC, Bertsch T, Fellner C, Djukic M, Sieber CC, et al. Sarcopenic obesity: Molecular clues to a better understanding of its pathogenesis? Biogerontology. 2015;**16**(1):15-29

[69] Morley JE. Hormones and sarcopenia. Current Pharmaceutical Design. 2017;**23**(30):4484-4492

[70] Shin MJ, Jeon YK, Kim IJ. Testosterone and sarcopenia. World Journal of Men's Health. 2018;**36**(3):192-198

[71] Nass R. Endocrinology and Metabolism Clinics of North America. 2013;**42**(2):187-199

[72] Bartke A. Growth hormone and aging: Updated review. World Journal of Mens Health. 2019;**37**(1):19-30

[73] Cleasby ME, Jamieson PM, Atherton PJ. Insulin resistance and sarcopenia: Mechanistic links between common co-morbidities. The Journal of Endocrinology. 2016;**229**(2):R67-R81

[74] Sato K, Iemitsu M. Exercise and sex steroid hormones in skeletal muscle. The Journal of Steroid Biochemistry and Molecular Biology. 2015;**145**:200-205

[75] Chen LY, Wu YH, Liu LK, Lee WJ, Hwang AC, Peng LN, et al. Association among serum insulin-like growth factor-1, frailty, muscle mass, bone mineral density, and physical performance among community-dwelling middle-aged and older adults in Taiwan. Rejuvenation Research. 2018;**21**(3):270-277

[76] Zembron-Lacny A, Dziubek W, Wolny-Rokicka E, Dabrowska G, Wozniewski M. The relation of inflammaging with skeletal muscle properties in elderly men. American Journal of Men's Health. 2019;**13**(2):1557988319841934

[77] Barclay RD, Burd NA, Tyler C, Tillin NA, Mackenzie RW. The role of the IGF-1 signaling cascade in

muscle protein synthesis and anabolic resistance in aging skeletal muscle. Frontiers in Nutrition. 2019;**6**:146

[78] Garcia M, Seelaender M, Sotiropoulos A, Coletti D, Lancha AH Jr. Vitamin D, muscle recovery, sarcopenia, cachexia, and muscle atrophy. Nutrition. 2019;**60**:66-69

[79] Chung E, Mo H, Wang S, Zu Y, Elfakhani M, et al. Potential roles of vitamin E in age-related changes in skeletal muscle health. Nutrition Research. 2018;**49**:23-36

Chapter 4

Clinical Relations of Sarcopenia

IGP Suka Aryana

Abstract

Sarcopenia is one of geriatric syndromes, characterized by decreased muscle mass accompanied by decreased muscle strength and/or performance. It is more prevalent with increase in age, and the prevalence depends on the criteria applied and the characteristic of the elderly. Sarcopenia has a higher risk of morbidity and mortality in elderly patients. The definition criteria of sarcopenia are still controversial, but diagnostic criteria from the Asian Working Group for Sarcopenia and the European Working Group on Sarcopenia in Older People (EWGSOP) are the most used criteria for clinical practice. Pathogenesis sarcopenia involved a multifactorial process and is divided into intrinsic and extrinsic factors. Risk factors for sarcopenia include constitutional factors, aging, lifestyle, changes in body condition, and chronic diseases. Based on that, sarcopenia is divided into primary and secondary sarcopenia. There are three stage of sarcopenia, which are pre-sarcopenia, sarcopenia, and severe sarcopenia. Nutrition and exercise are the two main pillars to manage sarcopenia.

Keywords: sarcopenia, elderly, clinical, muscle, morbidity

1. Introduction

The consequences of sarcopenia due to aging are often not getting noticed. Sarcopenia, which is characterized by decreased muscle mass accompanied by decreased muscle strength and/or performance, is often regarded as an ordinary physiological change due to aging. Muscles that have a mass of nearly 50% of the body mass are very important because besides serving as a body movement tool, they also are endocrine organs (secrete proteins called myokines that affect the metabolism of bodies systematically) and protective organs (counteract the negative effects of body fat). If muscle mass decreases, then the protective function of the body will be disrupted.

As age increases, the prevalence of sarcopenia also increases, where at an age of 65–70 years, the prevalence is between 13 and 24%, and at the age of more than 80 years, it is more than 50% [1]. The prevalence of sarcopenia based on gender at the age of 60–69 years is found in 10% of men and 8% of women, while in those over 80 years, it is in 40% of men and 18% of women [2]. The prevalence also differs based on the health-care setting. In acute care hospitals (age > 65 years), the prevalence is 10%. In long-term care facilities (age > 70 years), it is 33%, and in community-dwelling elderly (age ≥ 60 years), it is 29% [3]. It is difficult to obtain the typical prevalence of sarcopenia because it depends on the definition applied and characteristics of the elderly, but in the results from large-scale studies involving 1000 or more participants, the prevalence rate is estimated to be between 6 and 12% [4].

Sarcopenia is a risk factor for adverse outcomes in the elderly, including frailty, fractures, falls, and mortality. Sarcopenic elderly patients have a higher risk of cardiovascular death, especially patients with obesity. In cancer patients, sarcopenia reduces the survival rate [4, 5]. Sarcopenia is also associated with a large health expenditure which, in the USA (in 2000), is reported to be approximately $18.5 billion ($10.8 billion for men and $7.7 billion for women) [6].

This chapter will discuss mainly about the clinical relations of sarcopenia as well as its definition, pathogenesis, risk factors, diagnosis, stage, and its management.

2. Definition and terminology of sarcopenia

Sarcopenia is a syndrome characterized by progressive, complete loss of mass, strength, and/or skeletal muscle performance that is at risk of causing physical disability, low quality of life, and death [7]. Based on the Asian Working Group for Sarcopenia (AWGS), elderly with low muscle mass coupled with low grip strength and/or low walking speed are diagnosed with sarcopenia [8]. The rationalization of the use of muscle mass and strength separately on sarcopenia criteria is because muscle strength does not depend solely on muscle mass and the relationship between strength and muscle mass is not linear. Therefore, defining sarcopenia only from muscle mass considered is to be narrow and of limited clinical value [9].

Another opinion states that there is another term for stating muscle assessment, dynapenia. Dynapenia can be defined as a syndrome of loss of muscle strength related to age but not caused by neurological or muscular disease. In determining the mechanism of dynapenia, it is different from the mechanism of sarcopenia. The incidence of sarcopenia is determined by multifactorals characterized by a decrease in muscle mass, strength, and/or performance, while dynapenia is determined by only one factor, namely muscle weakness.

Muscle weakness is one of the factors involved in the etiology of dynapenia which causes functional limitations or physical disabilities. The determination of dynapenia starts with screening individuals over 60 years of age. For groups with high risk, knee extension strength assessment should be carried out to establish the diagnosis of dynapenia, while in the low-risk group it is recommended to take grip strength assessment measurements to confirm the results of the previous screening. Nevertheless, sarcopenia is more widely studied and discussed than dynapenia [10].

3. Pathogenesis of sarcopenia

There are several mechanisms involved in the progression of sarcopenia (**Figure 1**). These mechanisms involve protein synthesis, proteolysis, neuromuscular integrity, and mobility of nutritional status. In individuals with sarcopenia, various mechanisms may be involved and their contribution varies relative to time [7]. Walston also believes that there is a multifactorial process that triggers sarcopenia. These triggers include chronic illness, fat infiltration, physical inactivity, hormonal changes, energy, protein intake, oxidative stress, and inflammatory processes. The inflammatory process is recognized as a basic mechanism that results in the stimulation of muscle protein catabolism [11].

When viewed from simpler pathogenesis, sarcopenia is divided into two factors, namely intrinsic and extrinsic factors. Intrinsic factors consist of accumulation of pro-inflammatory cytokines, oxidative stress, mitochondrial dysfunction, insulin resistance, and disorders of motor neuron endplates. While extrinsic factors consist of radiation, nutrition, drugs consumed, smoking

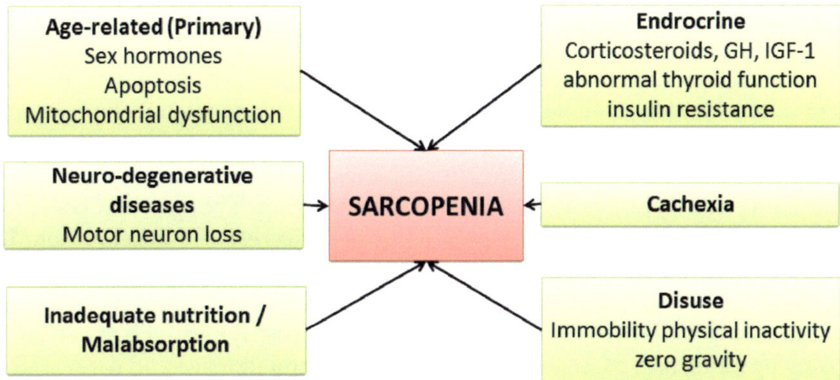

Figure 1.
Mechanisms of sarcopenia [7]. Note: Growth hormone (GH); insulin-like growth factor 1 (IGF-1).

behavior, infection, social environment, and physical activity. The interaction of intrinsic and extrinsic factors occurs in a complex, simultaneous, and dynamic manner. Every elderly person who experiences sarcopenia will have specific and individual interactions. In the end, the condition occurs as an imbalance of protein metabolism between degradation/catabolism and protein synthesis/anabolism. Sarcopenia occurs due to high protein catabolism accompanied by low protein anabolism [12]. High catabolism often results from chronic inflammation in the elderly. The elderly experience an immunosenescence condition that causes chronic inflammatory conditions of a low degree. In this condition, the body will be exposed to long-term pro-inflammatory cytokine mediators. Pro-inflammatory cytokines such as TNF-α will trigger muscle cell apoptosis in the elderly [13]. While protein metabolism decreases due to decreased protein intake and physical activity as well as decreased IGF-1 and growth hormone due to the process.

4. Risk factors for sarcopenia

Sarcopenia is a geriatric syndrome that is influenced by various factors including the following [7].

4.1 Constitutional factor

Constitutional factors are factors that are inherently closely related to humans, such as age, sex, and genetics. Age affects the occurrence of sarcopenia. The prevalence of sarcopenia increases with age, and even more than 45% of people over 80 years of age experience sarcopenia [14]. Decreased estrogen levels during menopause can cause a decrease in bone density, muscle mass, and muscle strength. In this case, the hormonal role of menopause is related to sarcopenia [15]. A study of 1971 elderly people in Kashiwa City, Chiba, Japan, showed differences in the prevalence of sarcopenia by sex, where in men it was 14.2%, while in women it was 22.1% [16]. Reverse results can be obtained elsewhere due to the differences in habits, activities, and nutritional intake. Several genes are related to lower limb muscle strength such as the growth differentiation factor 8 (GDF8) gene, cyclin-dependent kinase inhibitor 1 A (CDKN1A), and myogenic differentiation antigen 1 (MYOD1). Besides that, ciliary neurotrophic factor gene variant (CNTF A allele) is associated with loss of muscle strength [17].

4.2 Aging factor

The consequences of the aging process cause changes in the body system that is different for every human being. The aging process causes several changes in the human body system associated with sarcopenia, such as loss of neuromuscular function, changes in endocrine function, increased production of pro-inflammatory cytokines, and mitochondrial dysfunction. The aging process causes a decrease in the coordination of muscle work and a decrease in muscle strength due to a decrease in the number of alpha motor neurons and motor units. The aging process also results in atrophy of type II muscle fibers. Type II muscle fibers are found in large muscles that are important for basic activities such as getting up, going upstairs, and balance. Also, there is structural damage and decreased neuronal function at the motor center to the neuromuscular junction. Good muscle contraction requires the optimal functioning of the neuromuscular system because muscle tissue and nerve tissue are closely related to form motor neurons [18–20].

4.3 Lifestyle

The current lifestyle affects the incidence of sarcopenia in the elderly. Decreased food intake, especially protein, accompanied by less physical activity increases the risk of sarcopenia. Physical activity in the elderly experiences setbacks due to technological advancements such as elevators, escalators, vehicles, and others. Food consumption in the elderly is also changing, which tends to increase the consumption of fast food that is high in calories and fat. Optimal nutrition, especially protein, is needed to maintain muscle mass. Geriatric patients require a minimum of 1.2–2.0 g of protein/kilogram of body weight per day [21].

4.4 Changes in body condition

Prolonged bed rest increases the risk of sarcopenia. This is due to the lack of physical activity and mobility; immobility and underweight increase the risk of sarcopenia due to increased protein catabolism.

4.5 Chronic disease

Chronic diseases such as diabetes, advanced organ failure, cognitive impairment, and mood disorders cause chronic inflammation that can cause sarcopenia.

5. Diagnosis of sarcopenia

The diagnosis of sarcopenia is based on various risk factors reinforced by muscle weakness, fatigue, low endurance associated with decreased walking speed, impaired movement, and inability to perform daily tasks. The problem of diagnosis arises due to the variety of these sizes when viewed from age, race, and gender. There has not been much great research and precise accuracy to get a normal cutoff point. These sizes differ based on race and gender. Some researchers and research working groups also issued mixed figures.

Based on the European Working Group on Sarcopenia in Older People (EWGSOP), a criterion for sarcopenia is a loss of muscle mass coupled with one of the two conditions, namely loss of muscle strength and or loss of performance [7, 22]. In 2014, AWGS also issued a consensus with the same criteria with only changes in the size of the normal value. The other criteria for defining sarcopenia from the international society are listed in **Table 1**.

Study group	Definitions	Criteria		
		Muscle mass	Muscle strength	Performance
European Working Group on Sarcopenia in Older People [7]	Loss of muscle mass and strength	Low muscle mass (<2 SD below the mean of healthy young adults, aged 19–39 years)	Low handgrip strength (<2 SD below the mean of healthy young adults, aged 19–39 years)	Low gait speed (<2 SD below the mean of healthy young adults, aged 19–39 years)
Foundation for the National Institutes of Health Sarcopenia Project [23]	Loss of muscle mass and muscle weakness	Appendicular lean mass adjusted for body mass index <0.789 in men and < 0.512 in women	Handgrip strength <26 kg in men and < 16 kg in women	Gait speed ≤0.8 m/s
European Society for Clinical Nutrition and Metabolism (ESPEN) Special Interest Groups [24]	Loss of muscle mass and muscle strength	Low muscle mass (<2 SD below the mean in young adults, aged 19–39 years)	None	Reduced gait speed (<0.8 m/s in 4-min test) or reduced performance in any functional test used for comprehensive geriatric assessment
International Working Group on Sarcopenia [25]	Loss of muscle mass and function with age	Reduced muscle mass (appendicular lean mass relative to height squared ≤7.23 kg/m^2 in men and ≤ 5.67 kg/m^2 in women)	None	Gait speed <1 m/s
Society of Sarcopenia, Cachexia and Wasting Disorders [26]	Loss of muscle mass with reduced mobility	A lean appendicular mass relative to height squared (<2 SD below the mean of healthy young adults, aged 20–30 years)	None	Walking speed ≤1 m/s

Table 1.
Diagnostic criteria for sarcopenia from various international societies.

Sarcopenia measurement parameters consist of measurements of muscle mass, muscle strength, and function or physical performance (physical performance). In clinical practice, diagnosis can follow the algorithm set by AWGS in 2014, as shown in **Figure 2**. The normal threshold check requirements are clearly explained in **Table 2**. Experts often experience differences of opinion for difficulty in getting a normal value or cutoff and determining the best inspection technique to get the most accurate results.

5.1 Muscle mass

Measurement of muscle mass can be done by using computed tomography (CT), magnetic resonance imaging (MRI), and dual energy X-ray absorptiometry (DXA). The use of CT and MRI in muscle mass measurement is the measurement method that has the best accuracy because the measurement can distinguish fatty tissue from other soft tissues, but this measurement requires expensive costs [27]. Other measurements using DXA can provide results of body fat composition, bone

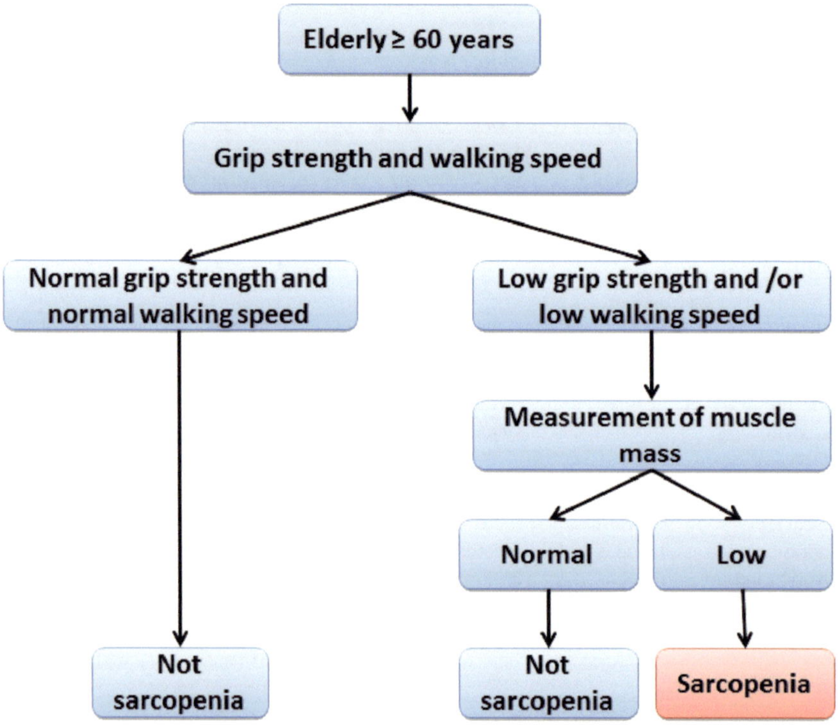

Figure 2.
Sarcopenia diagnosis algorithm based on the Asian working Group for Sarcopenia [8].

Criteria	Measuring instrument	Threshold
Muscle mass	DXA	
	• Man	<7.0 kg/m^2
	• Woman	<5.4 kg/m^2
	BIA	
	• Man	<7.0 kg/m^2
	• Woman	<5.7 kg/m^2
Muscle strength	Grip strength tests	
	• Man	<26 kg
	• Woman	<18 kg
Physical performance	Walking speed	<0.8 m/s

Table 2.
Measurement of sarcopenia according to the Asian working Group for Sarcopenia [8].

mineral, and fat-free body mass. The disadvantages of this technique are that the tools used are not portable [28]. While anthropometric measurements are very easy to do, it is not recommended to diagnose sarcopenia because it has a very high error rate. Anthropometric measurements are performed by measuring the circumference of the upper arm (LLA) or the circumference of the calf [27, 29]. Measurement of muscle mass is made using bio-impedance analysis (BIA), which is chosen for both research and clinical practice. Measurement using BIA has a good correlation value with MRI measurement in measuring body fat mass and body fat-free mass.

The most ideal muscle mass calculation for sarcopenia is based on the skeletal mass index (SMI), which is formulated by the appendicular skeletal mass (in kg) divided by height (in m^2). If there is a decrease in two deviations of muscle mass index/skeletal mass index (SMI) from the mean SMI population of young men and women, then it can be categorized as a decrease in muscle mass [7].

5.2 Muscle strength

Muscle strength can be measured in several ways, namely the grip strength test, knee extension test, and peak expiratory flow (PEF). The grip strength test is a simple examination so it is both used for clinical practice and research. Studies show this examination has a good correlation with inferior limb strength, mobility, and daily living activities (ADL). Examination of the knee extension is as good as a grip strength test, but this examination requires equipment and training in advance so it is not good for clinical practice. In peak expiratory flow (PEF) tests, it is very good for measuring respiratory muscle strength but cannot be used to measure the overall muscle strength [7]. The criterion for decreasing muscle strength according to the AWGS is less than 20 percentile of the mean population of grip strength tests [8].

5.3 Physical performance

An examination of physical performance is an examination of muscle function by performing physical activity. There are several ways of checking physical performance, such as the Short Physical Performance Battery (SPPB), walking speed, a 6-min walk test, time up and go test, and the strength of climbing stairs. Inspection with Short Physical Performance Battery (SPPB) is a standard inspection for physical performance. This check is carried out to evaluate balance, path, strength, and endurance. SPPB is done by assessing the ability to stand on both legs, in semi-tandem and tandem positions, the time needed to walk 8 ft, and the time

No	Component	Question	Answer
1	S = *Strength*	How difficult it is for the patient to lift or carry objects weighing 5 kg?	0 = No difficulties 1 = A little difficult 2 = Very difficult or cannot do without help
2	A = *Assistance walking*	How difficult is it for sufferers to walk across the room and do they need help?	0 = No difficulties 1 = A little difficult 2 = Very difficult, need help, or cannot do without help
3	R = *Rise from a chair*	How difficult it is for the sufferer to get up and move from a chair or bed?	0 = No difficulties 1 = A little difficult 2 = Very difficult, need help, or cannot do without help
4	C = *Climb stairs*	How difficult it is to the sufferer to climb 10 stairs?	0 = No difficulties 1 = A little difficult 2 = Very difficult or cannot do without help
5	F = *Falls*	How many times has the patient fallen in the past year?	0 = Not dropped in the past year 1 = Fell 1–3 times in the past year 2 = Fell 4 times in the past year

Table 3.
Strength, assistance walking, rise from a chair, climb stairs, and falls [34].

needed to get up from a seat and get back to sitting for as much as five cycles [30]. Based on AWGS recommendations, physical performance can be measured by a test of running as far as 5 m. Walking speed provides predictive value for the condition of disability and predicts the course of the disease [31, 32]. Time to get up and go test is a method of measuring physical performance in the elderly by using subjects rising from a chair, walking at a close range, returning, and sitting as before [33]. Stair climb power test is used as a method for assessing foot impairment. But the stair climb power test is only used for research [7].

Currently, there is a questionnaire for Strength, Assistance walking, Rise from a chair, Climb stairs, and Falls (SARC-F), which can be used to detect early sarcopenia quickly and it has high specifications. This is because the diagnosis of sarcopenia using the SARC-F questionnaire does not require certain other measurement tools. This criterion is subjective only by conducting careful and thorough interviews. The SARC-F questionnaire has a good specificity and sensitivity in identifying the presence of sarcopenia. The sarcopenia category is defined if the SARCF score > 4, as shown in **Table 3** [34].

6. Category and stage sarcopenia

Sarcopenia is a condition with many different causes and outcomes. In some individuals, a single cause of sarcopenia can be identified, but in other cases, clinicians can fail to identify the cause of sarcopenia. To facilitate clinical practice, sarcopenia is categorized into primary and secondary sarcopenia (**Table 4**). The etiology of sarcopenia can be multifactorial in the elderly, so there is a possibility that a person belongs to the primary, secondary, or both types of sarcopenia [7].

Sarcopenia stage is divided into three types based on the condition of muscle mass, muscle strength, and physical performance. The division of sarcopenia is seen in **Table 5**.

Primary sarcopenia • **Age-related sarcopenia**	No other cause evident except aging
Secondary sarcopenia • **Activity-related sarcopenia**	Can result from bed rest, sedentary lifestyle, deconditioning, or zero-gravity conditions
• **Disease-related sarcopenia**	Associated with advanced organ failure (heart, lung, liver, kidney, and brain), inflammatory disease, malignancy, or endocrine disease
• **Nutrition-related sarcopenia**	Results from inadequate dietary intake of energy and/or protein, as with malabsorption, gastrointestinal disorders, or use of medications that cause anorexia

Table 4.
Category of sarcopenia by cause [7].

Stage	Muscle mass	Muscle strength	Performance
Presarcopenia	Decreased		
Sarcopenia	Decreased	Decreased or normal	Decreased or normal
Severe sarcopenia	Decreased	Decreased	Decreased

Table 5.
Stage of sarcopenia [7].

7. Management of sarcopenia

Sarcopenia is a condition caused by a variety of complex factors. Therefore, a Geriatric Patient Full Assessment (P3G) for the management of sarcopenia should be carried out interdisciplinary with a focused and comprehensive intervention. P3G aims to improve physical and psychological patients, optimize drug administration to reduce the incidence of hospitalization and the risk of mortality, and increase patient satisfaction. P3G is carried out with an interdisciplinary team consisting of geriatric doctors, nurses, social workers, pharmacists, and physiotherapists who make plans for integrated care [17].

Diet control and physical training such as resistance training and stretching have a positive impact on sarcopenia associated with chronic diseases such as diabetes mellitus, hypertension, and coronary heart disease. Besides, psychological supportive therapy is needed for the management of sarcopenia because psychological factors of patients with sarcopenia are important in both prevention and recovery. Here are some recommendations for the management of sarcopenia [35]:

a. Multimodal therapy can be carried out with balanced energy and protein supplementation for the prevention and recovery of sarcopenia. The recommended total protein intake is 1–1.5 g/kg/day.

b. The recommended protein consumption is of good quality such as the amino acid leucine.

c. Creatine supplementation to enhance the physical exercise effects of sarcopenia patients.

d. Vitamin D supplementation with doses above 100 nmol/L. A dose of vitamin D is given up to 50,000 IU per week.

e. Resistance and aerobic exercise are done for 20–30 min, 3 times a week.

A protein diet is an important key needed to prevent a progressive reduction in muscle mass. Its mechanism of action is by preventing a negative nitrogen balance. The recommended diet for healthy people is 0.8 g/kg/day (RDA = recommended diet allowance). In the elderly >70 years, 40% of the protein diet is less than the RDA. In elderly patients with sarcopenia, the minimum recommended diet is according to the RDA (0.8) and will be increased to 1–1.5 g/kg/day by the increase in physical activity and comorbidities. Adequate protein intake in the elderly over 70 years has a positive effect on the ability to maintain muscle reserves and prevent sarcopenia. The positive effect is because the protein diet stimulates insulin-like growth factor 1 (IGF-1). Increased levels of IGF-1 as a result of this diet have an impact on preventing decreased protein synthesis and decreased muscle mass [36].

The use of creatine as a treatment for sarcopenia is still controversial because several studies have different results. In one study, the results showed that the elderly who took creatine supplements followed by endurance training experienced an increased muscle mass and strength. However, other studies show conflicting results, where creatine supplementation does not affect the muscle mass and strength [37].

Vitamin D levels can affect the incidence of sarcopenia. Some data show that inadequate levels of vitamin D can reduce muscle function and are associated with sarcopenia. Low levels of 25 (OH) D are associated with lower muscle mass, lower functional test results and can be used to predict muscle mass loss which will be one of the causes of disability. Lack of vitamin D is associated with poorer muscle function and loss of muscle mass [17].

Important physical activity becomes a pillar of conventional management that is very profitable. Large observational studies such as the British Regional Heart Study (BRHS), the Third National Health and Nutrition Examination Survey (NHANES III), and the Cardiovascular Health Study (CHS) show an inverse relationship between CRP concentration and physical activity in the elderly. The Health Aging and Body Composition (Health ABC) Study also found a linear tendency to decrease TNF with increased physical activity [9]. Therefore, physical activity is very necessary for the management of sarcopenia. The management of sarcopenia through physical activity must be designed with specific guidelines so that it gradually burdens muscles and makes positive adaptations. This should also be noted in physiology related to age and aging to avoid injury. Physical exercise in sarcopenia patients is focused on dynamic movements that target the major or major muscle groups such as knee and hip extensors through intrinsic and eccentric movements. The period of heating and cooling in the elderly is sought to last 15–20 min when heating and 10–15 min when cooling [38].

Management of other sarcopenia is still under studies, such as the therapeutic approach of using testosterone, estrogen, dehydroepiandrosterone (DHEA), and angiotensin-converting enzyme inhibitors (ACE inhibitors) [17].

8. Conclusions

Sarcopenia is more prevalent in older patients, especially men, and is defined by decreased muscle mass with decreased muscle strength and/or performance. Sarcopenia can cause multiple morbidities in the elderly, including frailty, fractures, falls, and even death. There are multifactorial factors (divided into intrinsic and extrinsic factors) that trigger sarcopenia, but the inflammatory process is recognized as a basic mechanism. Constitutional factors, aging, lifestyle, changes in body condition, and chronic diseases are considered as risk factors for sarcopenia in the elderly. Diagnostic criteria for sarcopenia are still under controversy since there is a variety of the component because it differs based on race and gender. Criteria from EWGSOP and AWGS are the most widely used. Currently, SARC-F questionnaires can detect early sarcopenia and have high specifications. In clinical practice, sarcopenia is categorized into primary and secondary sarcopenia and is divided into three stadiums, which are pre-sarcopenia, sarcopenia, and severe sarcopenia. Management of sarcopenia should be interdisciplinary with a focused and comprehensive intervention. Nutrition and physical training are the most important therapies for sarcopenia in the elderly.

Conflict of interest

The authors declare no conflict of interest.

Author details

IGP Suka Aryana
Geriatric Division, Internal Medicine Department, Medical Faculty of Udayana University, Sanglah Teaching Hospital, Bali, Indonesia

*Address all correspondence to: ptsuka_aryana@unud.ac.id

References

[1] Kim T, Choi KM. Sarcopenia: Definition, epidemiology, and pathophysiology. Journal of Bone Metabolism. 2013;**20**:1-10. DOI: 10.11005/jbm.2013.20.1.1

[2] Melton LJ, Khosla S, Crowson BS, O'Connor MK, O'Fallon WM, Riggs BL. Epidemiology of sarcopenia. Journal of the American Geriatrics Society. 2000;**48**(6):625-630. DOI: 10.1111/j.1532-5415.2000.tb04719.x

[3] Cruz-Jentoft AJ, Landi F, Schneider SM, Zuniga C, Arai H, Boirie Y, et al. Prevalence of and interventions for sarcopenia in ageing adults: A systematic review. Report of the international sarcopenia initiative (EWGSOP and IWGS). Age and Ageing. 2014;**43**(6):748-759. DOI: 10.1093/ageing/afu115

[4] Shimokata H, Shimada H, Satake S, Endo N, Shibasaki K, Ogawa S, et al. Chapter 2 epidemiology of sarcopenia. Geriatrics & Gerontology International. 2018;**18**(1):13-22. DOI: 10.1111/ggi.13320

[5] Dennison EM, Sayer AA, Cooper C. Epidemiology of sarcopenia and insight into possible therapeutic targets. Nature Reviews Rheumatology. 2017;**13**(6): 340-347. DOI: 10.1038/nrrheum.2017.60

[6] Janssen I, Shepard DS, Katzmarzyk PT, Roubenoff R. The healthcare costs of sarcopenia in the United States. Journal of the American Geriatrics Society. 2004;**52**:80-85. DOI: 10.1111/j.1532-5415.2004.52014.x

[7] Cruz-Jentoft AJ, Baeyens JP, Bauer JM, Boirie Y, Cederholm T, Landi F, et al. Sarcopenia: European consensus on definition and diagnosis. Age and Ageing. 2010;**39**(4):412-423. DOI: 10.1093/ageing/afq034

[8] Chen LK, Liu LK, Woo J, Assantachai P, Auyeung TW, Bahyah KS, et al. Sarcopenia in Asia: Consensus report of the Asian working group for sarcopenia. Journal of the American Medical Directors Association. 2014;**15**(2):95-101. DOI: 10.1016/j.jamda.2013.11.025

[9] Brandt C, Pedersen BK. The role of exercise-induced myokines in muscle homeostasis and the defense against chronic diseases. Journal of Biomedicine and Biotechnology. 2010;**1**:1-6. DOI: 10.1155/2010/520258

[10] Seene T, Kaasik P. Muscle weakness in the elderly: Role of sarcopenia, dynapenia, and possibilities for rehabilitation. European Review of Aging and Physical Activity. 2012;**9**:109-117. DOI: 10.1007/s11556-012-0102-8

[11] Walston JD. Sarcopenia in older adults. Current Opinion in Rheumatology. 2012;**24**(6):623-627. DOI: 10.1097/BOR.0b013e328358d59b

[12] Pedersen BK. The diseasome of physical inactivity and the role of myokines in muscle—Fat cross talk. The Journal of Physiology. 2009;**587**(3):5559-5568. DOI: 10.1113/jphysiol.2009.179515

[13] Marzetti E, Calvani R, Bernabei R, Leeuwenburgh C. Apoptosis in skeletal myocytes: A potential target for interventions against sarcopenia and physical frailty—A mini-review. Gerontology. 2012;**58**:99-106. DOI: 10.1159/000330064

[14] Moreira VG, Perez M, Lourenço RA. Prevalence of sarcopenia and its associated factors: The impact of muscle mass, gait speed, and handgrip strength reference values on reported frequencies. Clinics. 2019;**74**(7):1-7. DOI: 10.6061/clinics/2019/e477

[15] Messier V, Rabasa-lhoret R, Barbat-artigas S, Elisha B, Karelis AD,

Aubertin-Leheudre M. Maturitas menopause and sarcopenia: A potential role for sex hormones. Maturitas. 2011;**68**(4):331-336. DOI: 10.1016/j.maturitas.2011.01.014

[16] Ishii S, Tanaka T, Akishita M, Ouchi Y, Tuji T, Iijima K. Metabolic syndrome , sarcopenia and role of sex and age: Cross-sectional analysis of Kashiwa cohort study. PLOS One. 2011;**9**(11):1-8. DOI: 10.1371/journal.pone.0112718

[17] Setiati S, Rizka A. Sarkopenia. In: Setiati S, Alwi I, Sudoyo AW, Simadibrata MK, Setiyohadi B, Syam AF, editors. Buku Ajar Ilmu Penyakit Dalam. 6th ed. Jakarta: Balai Penerbit FKUI; 2014. pp. 3717-3724

[18] Puts MTE, Visser M, Twisk JWR, Deeg DJH, Lips P. Endocrine and inflammatory markers as predictors of frailty. Clinical Endocrinology. 2005;**63**(4):403-411. DOI: 10.1111/j.1365-2265.2005.02355.x

[19] Fried LP, Walston JD, Ferrucci L. Frailty. In: Halter JB, Ouslander JG, Tinetti ME, Studeenski S, High KP, Asthana S, editors. Hazzard's Geriatric Medicine and Gerontology. 6th ed. New York: McGraw Hill; 2009. pp. 631-645

[20] Yao X, Hamilton RG, Weng NP, Xue QL, Bream JH, Li H, et al. Frailty is associated with impairment of vaccine-induced antibody response and increase in post-vaccination influenza infection in community-dwelling older adults. Vaccine. 2011;**29**(31):5015-5021. DOI: 10.1016/j.vaccine.2011.04.077

[21] Baum JI, Kim IY, Wolfe RR. Protein consumption and the elderly: What is the optimal level of intake? Nutrients. 2016;**8**(6):1-9. DOI: 10.3390/nu8060359

[22] Giannoulis MG, Martin FC, Nair KS, Umpleby AM, Sonksen P. Hormone replacement therapy and physical function in healthy older men. Time to talk hormones? Endocrine Reviews. 2012;**33**(3):314-377. DOI: 10.1210/er.2012-1002

[23] Studenski SA et al. The FNIH sarcopenia project: Rationale, study description, conference recommendations and final estimates. The Journals of Gerontology. Series A, Biological Sciences and Medical Sciences. 2014;**69**:547-558. DOI: 10.1093/gerona/glu010

[24] Muscaritoli M et al. Consensus definition of sarcopenia, cachexia and pre-cachexia: Joint document elaborated by special interest groups (SIG) "cachexia-anorexia in chronic wasting diseases" and "nutrition in geriatrics". Clinical Nutrition. 2010;**29**:154-159. DOI: 10.1016/j.clnu.2009.12.004

[25] Fielding RA et al. International working group on sarcopenia sarcopenia: An undiagnosed condition in older adults. Current consensus definition: Prevalence, etiology, and consequences. Journal of the American Medical Directors Association. 2011;**12**:249-256. DOI: 10.1016/j.jamda.2011.01.003

[26] Morley JE et al. Sarcopenia with limited mobility: An international consensus. Journal of the American Medical Directors Association. 2011;**12**:403-409. DOI: 10.1016/j.jamda.2011.04.014

[27] Benton MJ, Whyte MD, Dyal BW. Sarcopenic obesity: Strategies for management. The American Journal of Nursing. 2011;**111**(12):38-44. DOI: 10.1097/01.NAJ.0000408184.21770.98

[28] Rubbieri G, Mossello E, Di Bari M. Techniques for the diagnosis of sarcopenia. Clinical Cases in Mineral and Bone Metabolism. 2014;**11**(3):181-184. DOI: 1138/ccmbm/2014.11.3.181

[29] Riyadi MA, Nugraha A, Santoso MB, Septaditya D, Prakoso T.

Development of bio-impedance analyzer (BIA) for body fat calculation. IOP Conference Series: Materials Science and Engineering. 2017;**190**:1. DOI: 10.1088/1757-899X/190/1/012018

[30] Ansai JH, Fernandes S, Oliveira T, Pretti F, Ferreira C, Lunardi AC, et al. Evolution of physical performance and handgrip strength in elderly assisted by an interdisciplinary domiciliary assistance program during one year. Fisioterapia e Pesquisa. 2013;**20**:197-202

[31] Perera S, Patel KV, Rosano C, Rubin SM, Satterfield S, Harris T, et al. Gait speed predicts incident disability: A pooled analysis. The Journals of Gerontology. Series A, Biological Sciences and Medical Sciences. 2015;**71**(1):63-71. DOI: 10.1093/gerona/glv126

[32] Rodríguez-Mañas L, Féart C, Mann G, Viña J, Chatterji S, Chodzko-Zajko W, et al. Searching for an operational definition of frailty: A delphi method based consensus statement. The frailty operative definition-consensus conference project. The Journals of Gerontology. Series A, Biological Sciences and Medical Sciences. 2013;**68**(1):62-67. DOI: 10.1093/gerona/gls119

[33] Ibrahim A, Singh DKA, Shahar S. 'Timed up and go' test: Age, gender and cognitive impairment stratified normative values of older adults. PLOS One. 2017;**12**(10):1-14. DOI: 10.1371/journal.pone.0185641

[34] Morley JE, Malmstrom TK, Miller DK. A simple frailty questionnaire (FRAIL) predicts outcomes in middle aged African Americans. The Journal of Nutrition, Health & Aging. 2012;**16**(7):601-608. DOI: 10.1007/s12603-012-0084-2

[35] Clegg A, Young J, Iliffe S, Rikkert MO, Rockwood K. Frailty in elderly people. The Lancet. 2013;**381**(9868):752-762. DOI: 10.1016/S0140-6736(12)62167-9

[36] Evenhuis HM, Hermans H, Hilgenkamp TIM, Bastiaanse LP, Echteld MA. Frailty and disability in older adults with intellectual disabilities: Results from the healthy ageing and intellectual disability study. Journal of the American Geriatrics Society. 2012;**60**(5):934-938. DOI: 10.1111/j.1532-5415.2012.03925.x

[37] Martone A, Lattanzio F, Abbatecola A, Carpia D, Tosato M, Marzetti E, et al. Treating sarcopenia in older and oldest old. Current Pharmaceutical Design. 2015;**21**(13):1715-1722. DOI: 10.2174/1381612821666150130122032

[38] Yu J. The etiology and exercise implications of sarcopenia in the elderly. International Journal of Nursing Sciences. 2015;**2**(2):199-203. DOI: 10.1016/j.ijnss.2015.04.010

Section 2

Prevention and Treatment of Muscular Atrophy

Chapter 5

Drugs for the Treatment of Muscle Atrophy

Linlin Chen, Hong Zhang, Mengyi Chi, Quanjun Yang and Cheng Guo

Abstract

Muscle mass is maintained through an interplay between anabolic and catabolic pathways. The ubiquitin-proteasome system plays an important role in the proteolysis progress during skeletal muscle atrophy which can be blocked by some proteasome inhibitors. But few studies have demonstrated the ability of these inhibitors to preserve muscle mass and architecture under catabolic condition in vivo. The insulin-like growth factor-1/phosphatidylinositide 3-kinases/protein kinase B/mammalian target of rapamycin (IGF-1/PI3K/Akt/mTOR) pathway was associated with anabolic pathways. The activation of IGF-1 causes muscle hypertrophy; however, it cannot be used as a drug target. Myostatin pathway maintains activation that can induce skeletal muscle atrophy involved with various transcriptional and genetic factors. Skeletal muscle atrophy is a debilitating consequence of multiple chronic diseases and conditions that involve starvation. It reduces treatment options and positive clinical outcomes as well as compromising quality of life and increasing morbidity and mortality. Though considerable research has been undertaken to find the drug target and the molecular mechanisms that improve skeletal muscle atrophy, no drug was approved to treat skeletal muscle atrophy. However, these years, the signaling pathways involved in muscle atrophy were clarified and some effective treatments were currently available to prevent, attenuate, or reverse muscle atrophy for experiment research.

Keywords: muscle atrophy, sarcopenia, cachexia, anabolic, catabolic

1. Introduction

The pathophysiology of skeletal muscle atrophy is multifactorial, with cancer, sepsis, renal and cardiac failure, acquired immune deficiency syndrome (AIDS) and chronic obstructive pulmonary disease (COPD) as well as inactivity or during aging [1–3]. These factors gradually lead to muscle wasting and weakness by decreasing protein synthesis and accelerating protein degradation, which are characterized by substantial decrease in myonuclear number, muscle fiber cross-sectional area, muscle strength and protein content while increasing in fatigability and resistance to insulin [4, 5]. Muscle atrophy is recognized as an independent predictor of mortality and is associated with functional impairment and poor quality of life [6].

Studies have revealed that different types of molecular mediators/catabolic players such as pro-inflammatory cytokines i.e. tumor necrosis factor-α (TNF-α), interleukin-6 (IL-6), interleukin-1 (IL-1), interferon gamma (IFN-γ) and

TNF-like weak inducer of apoptosis (TWEAK), eicosanoids and transforming growth factor-β (TGF-β) family effectors (such as activin A and myostatin) are involved in skeletal muscle atrophy under above mentioned clinical settings [7–9]. These cytokines binding to their respective receptor results in activation of several catabolic pathways including nuclear factor-kappa B (NF-κB), Janus kinase-signal transducer and activator of transcription (JAK-STAT) pathways and small mothers against decapentaplegic homolog 2/3 (SMAD2/3). In addition to cytokines, growth factors such as insulin-like growth factor-1 (IGF-1) signal through anabolic pathway (phosphatidylinositide 3-kinases/protein kinase B/mammalian target of rapamycin; PI3K/Akt/mTOR) to mediate functional repression of the transcription factors forkhead box protein O1 (FoxO1) or FoxO3 by inhibiting their nuclear translocation and overall levels, which together inhibit the transcription of muscle atrophy genes [10].

In spite of many promising therapeutic targets for improving skeletal muscle atrophy, no treatment has been successful to date. In this chapter, we classify the potential drugs currently in laboratory/preclinical research into four categories and then discuss their mechanism of action.

2. Anabolic medications

2.1 Androgen/androgen receptor modulators

Testosterone treatments increase muscle protein synthesis and fat free mass, and its effects on muscle are modulated by nutrition and exercise [11]. Several studies have shown the beneficial effects of testosterone supplementation on sarcopenia characteristics such as decreases in the muscle mass [12] and grip strength [13]. A study recently demonstrated that testosterone administration for 3 years in older men (over 60 years old) significantly improved stair-climbing power, muscle mass and power [14, 15]. Similarly, lower doses of testosterone supplementation in women with hysterectomy or chronic heart failure significantly increases lean body mass, 6-m walk time, chest press power and maximal voluntary contraction [16]. Evident showed that the effect of testosterone in improving skeletal muscle atrophy is related to the positive regulation of IGF-1 [12], wnt [17] and myostatin [18]. Although testosterone and its analogs can induce muscle growth and increase muscle strength [19], its clinical use is substantially limited by severe side effects including the increased risk of developing prostate hypertrophy, cancer, sleep apnea, masculinization, thrombosis complication and behavioral abnormalities [20, 21].

Compared with testosterone, the selective androgen receptor modulator (SARM) binds to androgen receptors with differing levels of sensitivity [22], showed androgenic effects in some tissues (such as muscle and bone), and has no effect on other organs (such as prostate or skin), thereby limiting adverse reactions such as prostate hypertrophy or androgen production. Enobosarm (GTx-024), an orally bioavailable nonsteroidal SARM, has been shown to increase lean body mass in phase I and II clinical trials of cancer cachexia patients [23, 24]. Moreover, the stimulation of reproductive organs with enobosarm seems to be less pronounced compared to testosterone administration. However, the phase III clinical trial of enobosarm failed to meet its common primary endpoint of preserving lean body mass and physical function [25]. Phase I clinical trials using another SARM non-steroidal oral preparation LGD-4033/VK5211 also showed increased muscle mass, but there was no effect on fat mass [26]. The 4-aza steroidal drug MK0773 (TFM-4AS-1) is a dual SARM and an inhibitor of 5α-reductase. Studies have shown that it can improve IGF-1 levels and muscle function in women, however, the trial was terminated due to increased cardiovascular risk [27]. GSK2881078, which is assessed for its impact on muscle growth and strength, has completed its phase I trial [28] and phase II trial for the treatment of weakness caused by COPD (NCT03359473). The development of SARM drugs still requires long-term follow-up and/or more effective and selective SARM trials to prove the safety and efficacy of SARM in improving physical function and health outcomes.

2.2 Ghrelin and its receptor agonist

Ghrelin is a growth hormone (GH)-releasing polypeptide that binds to the GH secretagogue receptor (GHSR-1α) and stimulates appetite by activating the neuropeptide Y (NY) in the hypothalamus and helps in regulation of body weight [29, 30]. Studies have shown that ghrelin can reduce dexamethasone, fasting, denervation, cancer and cisplatin-induced muscle atrophy [31, 32]. In cachexia induced by lung adenocarcinoma, ghrelin treatment can reduce the expression of TNF-α, IL-1β, IL-6 and C-reactive protein, and inhibit skeletal muscle atrophy by restoring the expressions of the p-Akt and p-FoxO1, and reducing the expressions of p-p38 mitogen-activated protein kinase and p-NF-κB in skeletal muscle of tumor-bearing mice [33]. A three-week clinical study of ghrelin therapy in cachexia patients with nausea, COPD and chronic heart failure (CHF) showed an increase in lean body mass and muscle strength [29, 34]. Although ghrelin plays a key role in stimulating appetite, gaining body weight and preventing muscle catabolism, its clinical efficacy is limited due to its half-life (0.5 h) and route of administration (intravenous) [35].

Ghrelin agonists (such as anamorelin) have the advantage of oral activity. Compared with ghrelin (0.5 h), it has a better half-life (7–12 h) [36]. A randomized, double-blind, placebo-controlled phase I clinical study showed that anamorelin gained body weight after 6 days of treatment [37]. In two phase II anamorelin trials in cachectic patients with advanced or incurable cancer [38] and two multinational phase III trials (ROMANA 1 and 2 trials) in cachectic patients with unresectable non-small cell lung cancer (NSCLC) [39], significant gains were recorded in lean body mass and body weight over 12 weeks, but there was no improvement in physical functions and hand-grip strength. Similarly, a multicenter, open-label, single-arm study investigated the efficacy and safety of anamorelin in advanced gastrointestinal cancer patients with cancer cachexia, and this study showed a positive effect of anamorelin on lean body mass, body weight, anorexia and patients' nutritional status [40]. Furthermore, anamorelin treatment was well tolerated over 12 weeks. Finally, two meta-analyses also strongly supported the positive effect of anamorelin on lean body mass and body weight [41, 42]. Recently, a single-center study on healthy young adults showed anamorelin elicited modest increases in hunger and achieved significant increases in hunger and caloric intake [43]. The findings are consistent with multi-center findings in cachectic cancer patients and expand the evidence supporting anamorelin as a potential intervention.

2.3 β-Adrenoceptor agonists

Muscle growth can also be stimulated by activation of G-protein coupled β2-adrenoreceptor (β2-AR), which causes protein kinase A activation [44] and thereby stimulating PI3K/Akt/mTOR signaling [45]. Formoterol is a β2-AR agonist, the administration of formoterol significantly increased the levels of follistatin and decreased the levels of myostatin and its receptors (activin receptor IIB, ActRIIB) in tumor-bearing rats, thereby regulating muscle mass loss [46, 47]. In addition to skeletal muscle, formoterol also shows a strong protective effect on the heart muscle [48]. Clinical studies have also shown that formoterol treatment can increase the content of PGC-1α and mtDNA in skeletal muscle of COPD patients to enhance the oxidation process of skeletal muscle and improve exercise ability [49]. Clenbuterol is another β2-AR agonist and can improve skeletal muscle atrophy in a variety of muscle atrophy models dominated by denervation [50], immobilization [51] and spinal cord injury [52]. However, due to concerns about potential cardiovascular side effects [44, 53], such as cardiac arrhythmia, there has been little interest in the clinical applications of β2-AR agonists for muscle atrophy treatment. Among them, espindolol may be a potentially attractive compound. It is a β1 receptor antagonist, a partial β2 receptor agonist and also has 5-HT1a receptor activities. In old rats, espindolol has been shown to significantly increase muscle mass, while reducing fat mass without negatively affecting heart function [54]. In addition, it has also shown very promising results in phase IIa cancer cachexia studies leading to increased muscle mass and grip strength [55, 56].

3. Enzyme inhibitors

3.1 Cox2 inhibitors

Cox2 is a bifunctional enzyme with cyclooxygenase and peroxidase activities. Cyclooxygenase activity is responsible for the synthesis of prostaglandins (PGE2) from arachidonic acid, while peroxidase activity can produce adjacent carcinogens. Both Cox2 and PGE2 are downstream effectors of cytokine activity and mediate cachexia [57]. A placebo-controlled study of celecoxib (Cox2 inhibitor) on cachectic patients with either head and neck or gastrointestinal cancer showed a significant increase of body mass and the quality of life [58]. In addition, a phase II non-randomized trial examined the efficacy and safety of celecoxib on cancer cachexia. Celecoxib administered at 300 mg/day for 4 months induced a significant increase of lean body mass, a decrease of serum TNF-α levels, and a trend toward a reduction of fatigue symptom [59]. Moreover, side effects such as grade 1/2 anemia, neuropathy and epigastralgia have been observed in only a few patients, and no grade 3/4 adverse events have been observed. Recently, a randomized double-blind clinical trial of combined treatment with megestrol acetate plus celecoxib versus megestrol acetate alone in cachexia-anorexia syndrome induced by gastrointestinal cancers was performed, however, this study failed to show that adding celecoxib (200 mg/day) to megestrol (320 mg/day) could enhance anti-cachexic effects of megestrol [60]. Meloxicam is another Cox2 inhibitor, and can suppress the expression of Cox2, Atrogin-1 and MuRF1 induced by lipopolysaccharide (LPS), and regulate the loss of muscle mass in rats by attenuating protein degradation [61]. In addition to cachexia, the administration of meloxicam can also inhibit the up-regulation of Atrogin-1 and MuRF1 in the muscles of arthritis rats and improve the loss of muscle mass [62].

3.2 Histone deacetylase inhibitors

Trichostatin A (TSA) is a well-known class I and II histone deacetylase inhibitor. Published data indicate that TSA regulates atrogenes level and controls muscle mass by reducing HDAC4 activity and myogenin expression, and increasing Dach2 level under denervation condition (neuromuscular disorders) [63]. TSA treatment can improve body weight, myofiber cross-sectional area and myofiber number [64]. Recent report shows that TSA inactivates FoxO by inhibiting HDAC activity, which leads to atrophy of skeletal muscle atrophy and contractile dysfunction [65]. In addition, under nutrition-deprived atrophy on C2C12 myotubes, TSA treatment leads to the suppression of FoxO target genes, including Lc3 (autophagy marker), MuRF1 and Atrogin-1 [66]. Similarly, TSA treatment can regulate muscle depletion by inhibiting the levels of Atrogin-1 and MuRF1 in dexamethasone-induced atrophic mice [63]. However, study shows that TSA treatment increased the expression level of follistatin (a negative regulator of skeletal muscle development), without retaining or increasing muscle mass in tumor-bearing mice [67]. Recent studies have shown that TSA can inhibit skeletal muscle atrophy and histomorphological alterations induced by unloading [68] and cigarette smoke (the main risk factor for COPD) [69]. Due to the contradictory findings, further research is needed to confirm the use of HDAC blockers to regulate atrophy.

3.3 PDE inhibitors

Torbafylline (HWA 448) is a xanthine derivative which acts as a phosphodiesterase (PDE) inhibitor [70]. Torbafylline treatment down-regulates the mRNA expression of cathepsin L, calpain and E3 ligases, and regulates the proteolytic pathway in burn-induced injury. In addition, the anti-atrophic effects of torbafylline have been demonstrated in casting, denervation or cancer induced cachexia models [70–72]. Torbafylline inhibits PDE activity leading to stimulation of the anti-proteolytic effect in PDE4/cAMP/Epac/PI3K/Akt pathway-mediated muscle atrophy [73]. Pentoxifylline (PTX) is another xanthine derivative that is non-selective in inhibiting PDE. Published data indicate that the administration of PTX under various pathological conditions in animal models (diabetes, tumors, sepsis) can stimulate the formation of cAMP, and by down-regulating calpain, cathepsin L and proteasome proteolytic system activity [74–76]. Other selective inhibitors of PDE, including rolipram and cilomilast have also been shown to reduce muscle atrophy in denervation and casting animal models [77, 78].

3.4 Angiotensin-converting enzyme inhibitors

ANGII induces muscle atrophy through several mechanisms including suppresses protein anabolism by reducing IGF-1 level and appetite, and promotes protein catabolism by increasing reactive oxygen species (ROS) and intermediate molecules (TNF-α, IL-6, glucocorticoids) in skeletal muscle [79]. In ACE-Is, enalapril treatment can reduce the risk of weight loss by>19% and delay the occurrence of cachexia by about 8 months [80]. Studies conducted in an old rat model show that the administration of enalapril can increase muscle strength and has a protective effect on age-related muscle degeneration [81]. Perindopril (an ACE inhibitor) has shown especially in a double-blind randomized controlled trial, which evaluated the effect of perindopril on the elderly 6-minute walking distance, thereby improving physical function, especially the 6-minute walk distance and reduced the incidence of hip fractures [82]. In subjects with dysfunction, perindopril improved exercise capacity to the extent reported after 6 months of exercise training [83]. However, the use of the perindopril in cachectic mice bearing colon-26 tumors to inhibit this pathway does not reduce muscle atrophy, nor does it increase the production of maximum muscle strength. Nonetheless, treatment with ACE inhibitors did enhance physical function and reduce fatigue of respiratory muscles. These effects appear to be due to a shift to a more oxidized muscle phenotype, as evident from increased oxidative enzyme capacity in the muscle cross-section [84].

4. Anti-inflammatory drugs

4.1 Thalidomide

Thalidomide is a glutamic acid derivative with various pharmacological activities, such as anti-inflammatory, immunomodulatory, anti-angiogenic, anti-emetic and sedative effects. Report shows that thalidomide and its derivatives can inhibit Cox2 and PGE2 synthesis induced by LPS in murine macrophages [85], and control systemic inflammation. In addition, evidence shows that thalidomide can reduce serum IL-6 and CRP levels in patients with cancer cachexia [86, 87]. Another study showed that thalidomide can maintain the fast-twitch type myofibers by reducing the expression of TNF-α and TGF-β1 in soleus muscle of cholangiocarcinoma rats [88]. Down-regulation of NF-κB/iNOS pathway by chronic thalidomide treatment improves hepatopulmonary syndrome and skeletal muscle atrophy in rats with biliary cirrhosis [89]. In addition to anti-inflammatory and anti-cachectic activity, thalidomide treatment (Phase II trial) also showed an effect on appetite in 64% of patients with advanced stage of cancer [87]. Studies reported that thalidomide (100 mg/day and 200 mg/day) treatment showed a significant improvement in body weight and skeletal muscle atrophy in AIDS associated cachexia patients [90]. Similarly, another research team worked with pancreatic cachexia patients and observed a significant increase in body weight of patients treated with thalidomide [91]. The lack of benefits was mainly due to the drug toxicity of thalidomide including peripheral neuropathy, dizziness, constipation and rash, considering that 47% of patients receiving active treatment were unable to continue taking thalidomide due to side effects and disease-related morbidity [92].

4.2 Anti-IL-6/STAT3

Evidence has shown that antibodies against IL-6 or its receptor can effectively reduce skeletal muscle atrophy and cachexia in mouse models [93, 94]. Preliminary results of a phase II double-blind trial in patients with advanced NSCLC have shown that ALD518 (humanized IL-6 monoclonal antibody) can reverse fatigue and prevent muscle loss [95]. Tocilizumab is an IL-6 receptor (IL-6R) neutralizing antibody approved by the FDA for rheumatoid arthritis. It can destroy the binding of IL-6/IL-6R to GP130, and cause the decrease of JAK/STAT3 pathway activity, reduce B cell hyperactivity and lead to a dramatic normalization of the acute phase reactions [96, 97]. Pharmacologic inhibition of the IL-6R using tocilizumab antennas skeletal muscle atrophy and function loss during infection [98]. Recently, a case of 65-year-old man who underwent percutaneous coronary intervention for acute myocardial infarction received tocilizumab led to prompt remission of Takayasu arteritis activity and improvement of left ventricular function and skeletal muscle atrophy [99]. Ruxolitinib, a JAK1/2 inhibitor, may protect muscle through on-target effects because it significantly reduces IL-6-induced STAT3 activation and myotube atrophy in vitro [100]. However, due to the inability to recruit qualified patients, the clinical trial of cancer patient study (NCT02072057) that investigating whether blocking downstream signaling of IL-6 by ruxolitinib improves muscle atrophy were terminated. In addition, there is evidence that C188-9 (a small molecule of STAT3 inhibitor) can reduce skeletal muscle atrophy in tumor-bearing mice [101, 102], but there are no relevant clinical studies.

4.3 Anti-TNF-α

Studies have shown that the administration of anti-murine TNF IgG in rats bearing Yoshida AH-130 ascites hepatoma can reduce circulating TNF-α and inhibit muscle protein degradation [103]. Similarly, injecting soluble TNF receptors (sTNFR1, a specific inhibitor of TNF-α) prevents the interaction of TNF-α with its receptor and attenuates ubiquitin transcription, reduce the waste of skeletal muscle and preserve body weight in cardiac cachexia [76]. A study reported the opposite effect of sTNFR1 on arthritic rat that it did not alter muscle mass and MuRF1 and Atrogin-1 gene expression [104]. Infliximab is a chimeric monoclonal antibody that blocks TNF-α action, thereby preventing its binding to cellular receptors and downstream immunological effects. A phase II study of the combined chemotherapy drugs gemcitabine and infliximab did not show the benefit of maintaining lean body mass or survival in pancreatic cancer cachexia patients [105]. Interestingly, in clinical trials of Crohn's disease patients with skeletal muscle atrophy or sarcopenia arising from chronic inflammation, significant gains were recorded in muscle volume and strength over 25 weeks of infliximab treatment [106, 107]. Etanercept is a recombinant fusion protein that acts as a decoy receptor to neutralize TNF-α, and has been used to treat inflammatory diseases including rheumatoid arthritis. In another study, significant weight gain was observed in rheumatoid arthritis patients who received etanercept twice a week for 12 consecutive months [108]. A phase I/II study compared the efficacy of etanercept with gemcitabine and gemcitabine alone for the treatment of advanced pancreatic cancer cachexia patients, and the results were also disappointing because the addition of etanercept did not improve symptoms of cancer cachexia [109].

4.4 Anti-IL-1α

MABp1 is a human antibody against IL-1α (a chronic inflammatory mediator) and has anti-tumor activity. Intravenous MABp1 treatment for 8 weeks in adults with metastatic solid cancer showed increased lean body mass and improved quality of life (fatigue, pain, and loss of appetite), and has no toxic; however, there was no control group in this study [110]. A randomized, double-blind, placebo-controlled phase III clinical study showed that MABp1 improved the lean body mass, anorexia, fatigue and pain scores in advanced colorectal cancer patients [111]. Another phase I dose-escalation study evaluating the IL-1α-targeted monoclonal antibody xilonix in patients with NSCLC showed increased lean body mass and improved symptoms, suggesting a clinically important response [112]. In view of this, a phase III placebo-controlled study of human antibodies against IL-1α has been conducted in patients with advanced colorectal cancer to assess the remission rate of the disease, muscle mass and appetite. Xilonix was very well tolerated by NSCLC patients, with the clinically significant reductions in pain, fatigue and improved lean body mass and appetite [113]. However, the primary limitation of this report is the small number of patients which made any comparisons statistically difficult.

4.5 TWEAK/Fn14 inhibition

The inflammatory cytokine TNF-like weak inducer of apoptosis (TWEAK) and its related receptor fibroblast growth factor-inducible 14 (Fn14) play multiple roles in proliferation, inflammation and wound repair. TWEAK/Fn14 signaling also negatively regulates muscle growth and function [8]. Report showed that TWEAK activates noncanonical NF-κB pathway and promotes myoblast fusion at low concentrations (10 or 100 ng/ml), and activates canonical NF-κB signaling to inhibit differentiation at high concentrations (500 ng/ml). Thus, TWEAK can maintain myoblast differentiation at physiological conditions; however, under pathological conditions (such as denervation and disuse), TWEAK/Fn14 system becomes activated and causes muscle atrophy [8]. Blocking antibodies against TWEAK antibody can improve muscle function in mice caused by myotonic dystrophy and amyotrophic lateral sclerosis (ALS) [114, 115]. Consistent with these findings, colon-26 tumor-bearing mice treated with anti-Fn14 antibodies showed increased weight and muscle mass, improved muscle fatigue, and increased survival [116]. These results indicate that neutralizing antibodies against TWEAK and Fn14 should be further explored in various muscle atrophy models and clinical trials.

5. Other investigational drugs

5.1 Myostatin inhibition

Existing evidence indicates that members of the TGF-β superfamily, such as myostatin and activin A, are powerful catabolic stimuli that can inhibit muscle growth and promote muscle protein loss in various disease states [117]. It is reported that myostatin can improve the dystrophy phenotype of mdx mouse models, sarcopenia in aging mouse models and muscle atrophy in tumor-bearing mice [118, 119], which can significantly inhibit systemic inflammation and prolong the survival of tumor-bearing mice without affecting tumor growth [117]. There are currently two main strategies for targeting myostatin signals: First, neutralize myostatin directly by using humanized myostatin antibody (LY2495655), and second, block ActRII by using soluble ActRIIB (ACE-031) or ActRII antibody (bimagrumab/BMY338). LY2495655 treatment had mixed results in elderly subjects: the appendicular lean body mass and gait speed were slightly improved, and despite increased muscle mass, grip strength was not affected [120]. However, a randomized, phase II trial in patients with pancreatic cancer, LY2495655 treatment have no significant improvement in muscle volume or functional. Additionally, among possibly drug-related adverse events, fatigue, diarrhea, and anorexia were more common in LY2495655-treated than in placebo-treated patients [121]. Soluble recombinant ActRIIB and other "ligand trap" interventions can generally inhibit TGF-β signaling and affect other tissues and processes, including reproduction and angiogenesis, with some causing severe off-target effects. Therefore, new strategies that target myostatin receptors and thereby reduce the activity of other ligands seem more promising. For example, after ACE-031 treatment, a group of 48 postmenopausal women gained weight and increased lean body mass [122]. However, in the phase II clinical trial conducted by ACE031 with Duchenne muscular dystrophy (DMD) patients and healthy volunteers, some participants experienced bleeding gums, nosebleeds, and skin vasodilation, which led to the interruption of the trial [123]. Blocking ActRII by administering BMY338 can greatly increase muscle mass and prevent dexamethasone-induced muscle atrophy in mice [124], and significantly improve patient's lean body mass, muscle mass, and 6-minute walking test in patients with myositis after 8 weeks of treatment. However, no significant differences were observed after 24 weeks of treatment [125]. In addition, there are no beneficial effects on these treatments were reported in cancer patients, while in COPD patients, muscle volume increases without affecting functional indicators, which is similar to the effect of BMY338 in sarcopenia patients [126, 127]. Therefore, these treatments seem to improve muscle mass and have less effect on muscle strength and other functional parameters [128].

5.2 Appetite stimulants

The FDA approved megestrol acetate (MA) as the treatment of cachexia caused by cancer and AIDS in 1993. More than 15 clinical trials have shown that this drug can significantly improve appetite and lean body mass at a dose of 160–1600 mg/day. MA can be used alone or as a supplement along with meloxicam in patients with cancer cachexia, showing a positive effect in controlling weight loss [129]. Although the mechanism of appetite stimulation/weight gain is unclear, studies have shown that it is related to the involvement of neuropeptide Y and the inhibition of pro-inflammatory cytokines such as IL-1, IL-6 and TNF-α [130, 131]. However, a newer meta-analysis started in 2015, which studied the use of non-cancer cachexia (HIV, COPD, renal failure and geriatric cachexia) and concluded that progesterone therapy (MA or medroxyprogesterone acetate) has a negligible effect on weight gain when treat of non-cancer cachexia [132]. MA treatment can also cause serious side effects such as thromboembolism, peripheral edema, hyperglycemia, hypertension, adrenal suppression and adrenal insufficiency [132].

Previous studies have shown that cannabinoids have the potential to improve appetite, body weight and fat mass, as well as amelioration of quality of life in several chronic diseases including cancer [133]. The results of a pilot study conducted in adult patients with advanced solid tumors showed that patients receiving delta-9-tetrahydrocannabinol (THC) treatment had a marked increase in appetite [134]. However, the study did not record changes in participants' body weight and lean body mass, and a larger trial was needed to study the effect of cannabinoids on skeletal muscle atrophy. A pilot study in patients with advanced NSCLC showed food intake and quality of life in patients treated with nabilone (a tetrahydrocannabinol) have improved significantly [135]. However, another randomized, double-blind placebo-controlled trial showed that nabilone did not improve the symptoms of nausea during radiotherapy in head and neck cancer patients, nor did it have significant benefits for the appetite and body weight [136].

5.3 Natural compounds

Recently, growing evidence has shown that natural products play a key role in the prevention and treatment of skeletal muscle atrophy. Numerous studies conducted in vitro and in vivo confirmed that resveratrol treatment can prevent proteolysis-inducing factor (PIF), angiotensin I and II, phorbol ester, 12-O-tetradecanoylphorbol 13-acetate (TPA), and dexamethasone-induced protein degradation [137]. In addition, resveratrol has been shown to protect muscle atrophy under various catabolic conditions, including cachexia and disuse [138, 139]. Salidroside is one of the main phenylpropane glycosides found in *Rhodiola rosea*. Research shows that salidroside treatment can effectively maintain body weight, reduce fat and gastrocnemius muscle loss in CT26 and LLC models. Additionally, in combination chemotherapy, salidroside can synergistically enhance the anti-tumor activity of cisplatin, especially reduce or eliminate cachexia caused by chemotherapy. Further analysis showed that salidroside can significantly increase the expression of p-mTOR and MyHC in the gastrocnemius muscle [140]. Matrine improves skeletal muscle atrophy in CT26 induced cachexia via inhibiting the production of TNF-α and IL-6 and activating the Akt/mTOR/FoxO3α signaling pathway [141]. Other natural medicines reported to improve skeletal muscle atrophy include imperatorin [142], parthenolide [143], ursolic acid [144] and cryptotanshinone [145], but more research is still needed to prove the anti-muscular atrophy effect of these compounds.

6. Conclusions

Up-regulation of muscle protein catabolic is a sign of atrophy, so most potential drugs target the proteolytic system to cure or prevent skeletal muscle atrophy.

Due to the multifactorial pathogenesis of muscle atrophy, combining new drugs with multimodal transport interventions including exercise methods and nutritional interventions may be the most promising approach; however, few clinical trials have investigated this approach. In this light, a better understanding of the contributing factors and underlying mechanisms of muscle atrophy is essential for the development of targeted therapies, and new methods of combination therapy for muscle atrophy treatment are needed.

Acknowledgements

This work was supported by the National Natural Science Foundation of China (No. 81873042 and 81872494).

Conflict of interest

The authors declare no conflict of financial interest.

Author details

Linlin Chen, Hong Zhang, Mengyi Chi, Quanjun Yang* and Cheng Guo*
Department of Pharmacy, Shanghai Sixth People's Hospital, Shanghai Jiao Tong University, Shanghai, China

*Address all correspondence to: myotime@sjt.edu.cn and guopharm@126.com

References

[1] Jackman RW, Kandarian SC. The molecular basis of skeletal muscle atrophy. American Journal of Physiology. Cell Physiology. 2004;**287**:C834-C843. DOI: 10.1152/ajpcell.00579.2003

[2] Lecker SH, Goldberg AL, Mitch WE. Protein degradation by the ubiquitin-proteasome pathway in normal and disease states. Journal of the American Society of Nephrology: JASN. 2006;**17**:1807-1819. DOI: 10.1681/asn.2006010083

[3] Scott D. Sarcopenia in older adults. Journal of Clinical Medicine. 2019;**8**: 1844. DOI: 10.3390/jcm8111844

[4] Dupont-Versteegden EE. Apoptosis in muscle atrophy: Relevance to sarcopenia. Experimental Gerontology. 2005;**40**:473-481. DOI: 10.1016/j.exger.2005.04.003

[5] Biolo G, Cederholm T, Muscaritoli M. Muscle contractile and metabolic dysfunction is a common feature of sarcopenia of aging and chronic diseases: From sarcopenic obesity to cachexia. Clinical Nutrition (Edinburgh, Scotland). 2014;**33**:737-748. DOI: 10.1016/j.clnu.2014.03.007

[6] Fearon K, Strasser F, Anker SD, et al. Definition and classification of cancer cachexia: An international consensus. The Lancet Oncology. 2011;**12**:489-495. DOI: 10.1016/s1470-2045(10)70218-7

[7] Llovera M, Carbó N, López-Soriano J, et al. Different cytokines modulate ubiquitin gene expression in rat skeletal muscle. Cancer Letters. 1998;**133**:83-87. DOI: 10.1016/s0304-3835(98)00216-x

[8] Mittal A, Bhatnagar S, Kumar A, et al. The TWEAK-Fn14 system is a critical regulator of denervation-induced skeletal muscle atrophy in mice. The Journal of Cell Biology. 2010;**188**:833-849. DOI: 10.1083/jcb.200909117

[9] Frost RA, Lang CH. Protein kinase B/Akt: A nexus of growth factor and cytokine signaling in determining muscle mass. Journal of Applied Physiology (Bethesda, MD: 1985). 2007;**103**:378-387. DOI: 10.1152/japplphysiol.00089.2007

[10] Schiaffino S, Dyar KA, Ciciliot S, Blaauw B, Sandri M. Mechanisms regulating skeletal muscle growth and atrophy. The FEBS Journal. 2013;**280**:4294-4314. DOI: 10.1111/febs.12253

[11] Bhasin S, Woodhouse L, Storer TW. Proof of the effect of testosterone on skeletal muscle. The Journal of Endocrinology. 2001;**170**:27-38. DOI: 10.1677/joe.0.1700027

[12] Ferrando AA, Sheffield-Moore M, Yeckel CW, et al. Testosterone administration to older men improves muscle function: Molecular and physiological mechanisms. American Journal of Physiology. Endocrinology and Metabolism. 2002;**282**:E601-E607. DOI: 10.1152/ajpendo.00362.2001

[13] Bakhshi V, Elliott M, Gentili A, Godschalk M, Mulligan T. Testosterone improves rehabilitation outcomes in ill older men. Journal of the American Geriatrics Society. 2000;**48**:550-553. DOI: 10.1111/j.1532-5415.2000.tb05002.x

[14] Storer TW, Basaria S, Traustadottir T, et al. Effects of testosterone supplementation for 3 years on muscle performance and physical function in older men. The Journal of Clinical Endocrinology and Metabolism. 2017;**102**:583-593. DOI: 10.1210/jc.2016-2771

[15] Iellamo F, Volterrani M, Caminiti G, et al. Testosterone therapy in women with chronic heart failure: A pilot double-blind, randomized, placebo-controlled study. Journal of the American College of Cardiology. 2010;**56**:1310-1316. DOI: 10.1016/j.jacc.2010.03.090

[16] Huang G, Basaria S, Travison TG, et al. Testosterone dose-response relationships in hysterectomized women with or without oophorectomy: Effects on sexual function, body composition, muscle performance and physical function in a randomized trial. Menopause (New York, NY). 2014;**21**:612-623. DOI: 10.1097/gme.0000000000000093

[17] Singh R, Bhasin S, Braga M, et al. Regulation of myogenic differentiation by androgens: Cross talk between androgen receptor/beta-catenin and follistatin/transforming growth factor-beta signaling pathways. Endocrinology. 2009;**150**:1259-1268. DOI: 10.1210/en.2008-0858

[18] Mendler L, Baka Z, Kovács-Simon A, Dux L. Androgens negatively regulate myostatin expression in an androgen-dependent skeletal muscle. Biochemical and Biophysical Research Communications. 2007;**361**:237-242. DOI: 10.1016/j.bbrc.2007.07.023

[19] Ferrando AA, Sheffield-Moore M, Paddon-Jones D, Wolfe RR, Urban RJ. Differential anabolic effects of testosterone and amino acid feeding in older men. The Journal of Clinical Endocrinology and Metabolism. 2003;**88**:358-362. DOI: 10.1210/jc.2002-021041

[20] Khoo TK. Adverse events associated with testosterone administration. The New England Journal of Medicine. 2010;**363**:1865-1866; author reply 1866-1867. DOI: 10.1056/NEJMc1009326

[21] Curran MJ, Bihrle W III. Dramatic rise in prostate-specific antigen after androgen replacement in a hypogonadal man with occult adenocarcinoma of the prostate. Urology. 1999;**53**:423-424. DOI: 10.1016/s0090-4295(98)00348-3

[22] Mohler ML, Bohl CE, Jones A, et al. Nonsteroidal selective androgen receptor modulators (SARMs): Dissociating the anabolic and androgenic activities of the androgen receptor for therapeutic benefit. Journal of Medicinal Chemistry. 2009;**52**:3597-3617. DOI: 10.1021/jm900280m

[23] Kim J, Wu D, Hwang DJ, Miller DD, Dalton JT. The para substituent of S-3-(phenoxy)-2-hydroxy-2-methyl-N-(4-nitro-3-trifluoromethyl-phenyl)-propionamides is a major structural determinant of in vivo disposition and activity of selective androgen receptor modulators. The Journal of Pharmacology and Experimental Therapeutics. 2005;**315**:230-239. DOI: 10.1124/jpet.105.088344

[24] Dobs AS, Boccia RV, Croot CC, et al. Effects of enobosarm on muscle wasting and physical function in patients with cancer: A double-blind, randomised controlled phase 2 trial. The Lancet Oncology. 2013;**14**:335-345. DOI: 10.1016/s1470-2045(13)70055-x

[25] Crawford J, Prado CM, Johnston MA, et al. Study design and rationale for the phase 3 clinical development program of enobosarm, a selective androgen receptor modulator, for the prevention and treatment of muscle wasting in cancer patients (POWER trials). Current Oncology Reports. 2016;**18**:37. DOI: 10.1007/s11912-016-0522-0

[26] Basaria S, Collins L, Dillon EL, et al. The safety, pharmacokinetics, and effects of LGD-4033, a novel nonsteroidal oral, selective androgen receptor modulator, in healthy young men. The Journals of Gerontology Series A Biological Sciences and Medical Sciences. 2013;**68**:87-95. DOI: 10.1093/gerona/gls078

[27] Papanicolaou DA, Ather SN, Zhu H, et al. A phase IIA randomized, placebo-controlled clinical trial to study the efficacy and safety of the selective androgen receptor modulator (SARM), MK-0773 in female participants with sarcopenia. The Journal of Nutrition, Health and Aging. 2013;**17**:533-543. DOI: 10.1007/s12603-013-0335-x

[28] Neil D, Clark RV, Magee M, et al. GSK2881078, a SARM, produces dose-dependent increases in lean mass in healthy older men and women. The Journal of Clinical Endocrinology and Metabolism. 2018;**103**:3215-3224. DOI: 10.1210/jc.2017-02644

[29] Nagaya N, Itoh T, Murakami S, et al. Treatment of cachexia with ghrelin in patients with COPD. Chest. 2005;**128**:1187-1193. DOI: 10.1378/chest.128.3.1187

[30] Barazzoni R, Zhu X, Deboer M, et al. Combined effects of ghrelin and higher food intake enhance skeletal muscle mitochondrial oxidative capacity and AKT phosphorylation in rats with chronic kidney disease. Kidney International. 2010;**77**:23-28. DOI: 10.1038/ki.2009.411

[31] Porporato PE, Filigheddu N, Reano S, et al. Acylated and unacylated ghrelin impair skeletal muscle atrophy in mice. The Journal of Clinical Investigation. 2013;**123**:611-622. DOI: 10.1172/jci39920

[32] Chen JA, Splenser A, Guillory B, et al. Ghrelin prevents tumour- and cisplatin-induced muscle wasting: Characterization of multiple mechanisms involved. Journal of Cachexia, Sarcopenia and Muscle. 2015;**6**:132-143. DOI: 10.1002/jcsm.12023

[33] Tsubouchi H, Yanagi S, Miura A, Matsumoto N, Kangawa K, Nakazato M. Ghrelin relieves cancer cachexia associated with the development of lung adenocarcinoma in mice. European Journal of Pharmacology. 2014;**743**:1-10. DOI: 10.1016/j.ejphar.2014.09.025

[34] Nagaya N, Moriya J, Yasumura Y, et al. Effects of ghrelin administration on left ventricular function, exercise capacity, and muscle wasting in patients with chronic heart failure. Circulation. 2004;**110**:3674-3679. DOI: 10.1161/01.Cir.0000149746.62908.Bb

[35] Strasser F, Lutz TA, Maeder MT, et al. Safety, tolerability and pharmacokinetics of intravenous ghrelin for cancer-related anorexia/cachexia: A randomised, placebo-controlled, double-blind, double-crossover study. British Journal of Cancer. 2008;**98**:300-308. DOI: 10.1038/sj.bjc.6604148

[36] Pietra C, Takeda Y, Tazawa-Ogata N, et al. Anamorelin HCl (ONO-7643), a novel ghrelin receptor agonist, for the treatment of cancer anorexia-cachexia syndrome: Preclinical profile. Journal of Cachexia, Sarcopenia and Muscle. 2014;**5**:329-337. DOI: 10.1007/s13539-014-0159-5

[37] Garcia JM, Friend J, Allen S. Therapeutic potential of anamorelin, a novel, oral ghrelin mimetic, in patients with cancer-related cachexia: A multicenter, randomized, double-blind, crossover, pilot study. Supportive Care in Cancer: Official Journal of the Multinational Association of Supportive Care in Cancer. 2013;**21**:129-137. DOI: 10.1007/s00520-012-1500-1

[38] Garcia JM, Boccia RV, Graham CD, et al. Anamorelin for patients with cancer cachexia: An integrated analysis of two phase 2, randomised, placebo-controlled, double-blind trials. The Lancet Oncology. 2015;**16**:108-116. DOI: 10.1016/s1470-2045(14)71154-4

[39] Temel JS, Abernethy AP, Currow DC, et al. Anamorelin in patients with non-small-cell lung cancer and cachexia (ROMANA

1 and ROMANA 2): Results from two randomised, double-blind, phase 3 trials. The Lancet Oncology. 2016;**17**:519-531. DOI: 10.1016/s1470-2045(15)00558-6

[40] Hamauchi S, Furuse J, Takano T, et al. A multicenter, open-label, single-arm study of anamorelin (ONO-7643) in advanced gastrointestinal cancer patients with cancer cachexia. Cancer. 2019;**125**:4294-4302. DOI: 10.1002/cncr.32406

[41] Nishie K, Yamamoto S, Nagata C, Koizumi T, Hanaoka M. Anamorelin for advanced non-small-cell lung cancer with cachexia: Systematic review and meta-analysis. Lung Cancer (Amsterdam, Netherlands). 2017;**112**:25-34. DOI: 10.1016/j.lungcan.2017.07.023

[42] Bai Y, Hu Y, Zhao Y, et al. Anamorelin for cancer anorexia-cachexia syndrome: A systematic review and meta-analysis. Supportive Care in Cancer: Official Journal of the Multinational Association of Supportive Care in Cancer. 2017;**25**:1651-1659. DOI: 10.1007/s00520-016-3560-0

[43] Blum RA, Mair S, Duus EM. Appetite and food intake results from phase I studies of anamorelin. Journal of Cachexia, Sarcopenia and Muscle. 2019;**10**:1027-1035. DOI: 10.1002/jcsm.12439

[44] Lynch GS, Ryall JG. Role of beta-adrenoceptor signaling in skeletal muscle: Implications for muscle wasting and disease. Physiological Reviews. 2008;**88**:729-767. DOI: 10.1152/physrev.00028.2007

[45] Sandri M. Signaling in muscle atrophy and hypertrophy. Physiology (Bethesda, Md.). 2008;**23**:160-170. DOI: 10.1152/physiol.00041.2007

[46] Quanjun Y, Genjin Y, Lili W, et al. Serum metabolic profiles reveal the effect of formoterol on cachexia in tumor-bearing mice. Molecular BioSystems. 2013;**9**:3015-3025. DOI: 10.1039/c3mb70134d

[47] Busquets S, Toledo M, Marmonti E, et al. Formoterol treatment downregulates the myostatin system in skeletal muscle of cachectic tumour-bearing rats. Oncology Letters. 2012;**3**:185-189. DOI: 10.3892/ol.2011.442

[48] Toledo M, Springer J, Busquets S, et al. Formoterol in the treatment of experimental cancer cachexia: Effects on heart function. Journal of Cachexia, Sarcopenia and Muscle. 2014;**5**:315-320. DOI: 10.1007/s13539-014-0153-y

[49] D'Agostino B, Polverino M, Cirino G, et al. Exercise capacity and cytochrome oxidase activity in muscle mitochondria of COPD patients. Respiratory Medicine. 2010;**104**:83-90. DOI: 10.1016/j.rmed.2009.07.016

[50] Gonçalves DA, Silveira WA, Lira EC, et al. Clenbuterol suppresses proteasomal and lysosomal proteolysis and atrophy-related genes in denervated rat soleus muscles independently of Akt. American Journal of Physiology. Endocrinology and Metabolism. 2012;**302**:E123-E133. DOI: 10.1152/ajpendo.00188.2011

[51] Suzuki H, Yoshikawa Y, Tsujimoto H, Kitaura T, Muraoka I. Clenbuterol accelerates recovery after immobilization-induced atrophy of rat hindlimb muscle. Acta Histochemica. 2020;**122**:151453. DOI: 10.1016/j.acthis.2019.151453

[52] Ung RV, Rouleau P, Guertin PA. Functional and physiological effects of treadmill training induced by buspirone, carbidopa, and L-DOPA in clenbuterol-treated paraplegic mice. Neurorehabilitation and Neural Repair. 2012;**26**:385-394. DOI: 10.1177/1545968311427042

[53] Brett J, Dawson AH, Brown JA. Clenbuterol toxicity: A NSW poisons information centre experience. The Medical Journal of Australia. 2014;**200**:219-221. DOI: 10.5694/mja13.10982

[54] Pötsch MS, Tschirner A, Palus S, et al. The anabolic catabolic transforming agent (ACTA) espindolol increases muscle mass and decreases fat mass in old rats. Journal of Cachexia, Sarcopenia and Muscle. 2014;**5**:149-158. DOI: 10.1007/s13539-013-0125-7

[55] Lainscak M, Laviano A. ACT-ONE - ACTION at last on cancer cachexia by adapting a novel action beta-blocker. Journal of Cachexia, Sarcopenia and Muscle. 2016;**7**:400-402. DOI: 10.1002/jcsm.12136

[56] Stewart Coats AJ, Ho GF, Prabhash K, et al. Espindolol for the treatment and prevention of cachexia in patients with stage III/IV non-small cell lung cancer or colorectal cancer: A randomized, double-blind, placebo-controlled, international multicentre phase II study (the ACT-ONE trial). Journal of Cachexia, Sarcopenia and Muscle. 2016;**7**:355-365. DOI: 10.1002/jcsm.12126

[57] Baumgarten AJ, Fiebig HH, Burger AM. Molecular analysis of xenograft models of human cancer cachexia--Possibilities for therapeutic intervention. Cancer Genomics & Proteomics. 2007;**4**:223-231

[58] Lai V, George J, Richey L, et al. Results of a pilot study of the effects of celecoxib on cancer cachexia in patients with cancer of the head, neck, and gastrointestinal tract. Head & Neck. 2008;**30**:67-74. DOI: 10.1002/hed.20662

[59] Mantovani G, Macciò A, Madeddu C, et al. Phase II nonrandomized study of the efficacy and safety of COX-2 inhibitor celecoxib on patients with cancer cachexia. Journal of Molecular Medicine (Berlin, Germany). 2010;**88**:85-92. DOI: 10.1007/s00109-009-0547-z

[60] Kouchaki B, Janbabai G, Alipour A, Ala S, Borhani S, Salehifar E. Randomized double-blind clinical trial of combined treatment with megestrol acetate plus celecoxib versus megestrol acetate alone in cachexia-anorexia syndrome induced by GI cancers. Supportive Care in Cancer: Official Journal of the Multinational Association of Supportive Care in Cancer. 2018;**26**:2479-2489. DOI: 10.1007/s00520-018-4047-y

[61] Martin AI, Nieto-Bona MP, Castillero E, et al. Effect of cyclooxygenase-2 inhibition by meloxicam, on atrogin-1 and myogenic regulatory factors in skeletal muscle of rats injected with endotoxin. Journal of Physiology and Pharmacology: An Official Journal of the Polish Physiological Society. 2012;**63**:649-659

[62] Granado M, Martín AI, Villanúa MA, López-Calderón A. Experimental arthritis inhibits the insulin-like growth factor-I axis and induces muscle wasting through cyclooxygenase-2 activation. American Journal of Physiology. Endocrinology and Metabolism. 2007;**292**:E1656-E1665. DOI: 10.1152/ajpendo.00502.2006

[63] Bricceno KV, Sampognaro PJ, Van Meerbeke JP, Sumner CJ, Fischbeck KH, Burnett BG. Histone deacetylase inhibition suppresses myogenin-dependent atrogene activation in spinal muscular atrophy mice. Human Molecular Genetics. 2012;**21**:4448-4459. DOI: 10.1093/hmg/dds286

[64] Avila AM, Burnett BG, Taye AA, et al. Trichostatin A increases SMN expression and survival in a mouse model of spinal muscular atrophy. The Journal of Clinical Investigation. 2007;**117**:659-671. DOI: 10.1172/jci29562

[65] Beharry AW, Sandesara PB, Roberts BM, Ferreira LF, Senf SM, Judge AR. HDAC1 activates FoxO and is both sufficient and required for skeletal muscle atrophy. Journal of Cell Science. 2014;**127**:1441-1453. DOI: 10.1242/jcs.136390

[66] Tang H, Goldman D. Activity-dependent gene regulation in skeletal muscle is mediated by a histone deacetylase (HDAC)-Dach2-myogenin signal transduction cascade. Proceedings of the National Academy of Sciences of the United States of America. 2006;**103**:16977-16982. DOI: 10.1073/pnas.0601565103

[67] Bonetto A, Penna F, Minero VG, et al. Deacetylase inhibitors modulate the myostatin/follistatin axis without improving cachexia in tumor-bearing mice. Current Cancer Drug Targets. 2009;**9**:608-616. DOI: 10.2174/156800909789057015

[68] Dupré-Aucouturier S, Castells J, Freyssenet D, Desplanches D. Trichostatin A, a histone deacetylase inhibitor, modulates unloaded-induced skeletal muscle atrophy. Journal of Applied Physiology (Bethesda, MD: 1985). 2015;**119**:342-351. DOI: 10.1152/japplphysiol.01031.2014

[69] Ding J, Li F, Cong Y, et al. Trichostatin A inhibits skeletal muscle atrophy induced by cigarette smoke exposure in mice. Life Sciences. 2019;**235**:116800. DOI: 10.1016/j.lfs.2019.116800

[70] Combaret L, Tilignac T, Claustre A, et al. Torbafylline (HWA 448) inhibits enhanced skeletal muscle ubiquitin-proteasome-dependent proteolysis in cancer and septic rats. The Biochemical Journal. 2002;**361**:185-192. DOI: 10.1042/0264-6021:3610185

[71] Breuillé D, Farge MC, Rosé F, Arnal M, Attaix D, Obled C. Pentoxifylline decreases body weight loss and muscle protein wasting characteristics of sepsis. The American Journal of Physiology. 1993;**265**:E660-E666. DOI: 10.1152/ajpendo.1993.265.4.E660

[72] Baviera AM, Zanon NM, Carvalho Navegantes LC, Migliorini RH, do Carmo Kettelhut I. Pentoxifylline inhibits Ca^{2+}-dependent and ATP proteasome-dependent proteolysis in skeletal muscle from acutely diabetic rats. American Journal of Physiology. Endocrinology and Metabolism. 2007;**292**:E702-E708. DOI: 10.1152/ajpendo.00147.2006

[73] Joshi R, Kadeer N, Sheriff S, Friend LA, James JH, Balasubramaniam A. Phosphodiesterase (PDE) inhibitor torbafylline (HWA 448) attenuates burn-induced rat skeletal muscle proteolysis through the PDE4/cAMP/EPAC/PI3K/Akt pathway. Molecular and Cellular Endocrinology. 2014;**393**:152-163. DOI: 10.1016/j.mce.2014.06.012

[74] Arcaro CA, Assis RP, Zanon NM, et al. Involvement of cAMP/EPAC/Akt signaling in the antiproteolytic effects of pentoxifylline on skeletal muscles of diabetic rats. Journal of Applied Physiology (Bethesda, MD: 1985). 2018;**124**:704-716. DOI: 10.1152/japplphysiol.00499.2017

[75] Deval C, Mordier S, Obled C, et al. Identification of cathepsin L as a differentially expressed message associated with skeletal muscle wasting. The Biochemical Journal. 2001;**360**:143-150. DOI: 10.1042/0264-6021:3600143

[76] Steffen BT, Lees SJ, Booth FW. Anti-TNF treatment reduces rat skeletal muscle wasting in monocrotaline-induced cardiac cachexia. Journal of Applied Physiology (Bethesda, MD: 1985). 2008;**105**:1950-1958. DOI: 10.1152/japplphysiol.90884.2008

[77] Lira EC, Gonçalves DA, Parreiras ESLT, Zanon NM, Kettelhut IC, Navegantes LC. Phosphodiesterase-4 inhibition reduces proteolysis and atrogenes expression in rat skeletal muscles. Muscle & Nerve. 2011;**44**:371-381. DOI: 10.1002/mus.22066

[78] Hinkle RT, Dolan E, Cody DB, Bauer MB, Isfort RJ. Phosphodiesterase 4 inhibition reduces skeletal muscle atrophy. Muscle & Nerve. 2005;**32**:775-781. DOI: 10.1002/mus.20416

[79] Kackstein K, Teren A, Matsumoto Y, et al. Impact of angiotensin II on skeletal muscle metabolism and function in mice: Contribution of IGF-1, Sirtuin-1 and PGC-1α. Acta Histochemica. 2013;**115**:363-370. DOI: 10.1016/j.acthis.2012.09.009

[80] Anker SD, Negassa A, Coats AJ, et al. Prognostic importance of weight loss in chronic heart failure and the effect of treatment with angiotensin-converting-enzyme inhibitors: An observational study. Lancet (London, England). 2003;**361**:1077-1083. DOI: 10.1016/s0140-6736(03)12892-9

[81] Marzetti E, Calvani R, DuPree J, et al. Late-life enalapril administration induces nitric oxide-dependent and independent metabolic adaptations in the rat skeletal muscle. Age (Dordrecht, Netherlands). 2013;**35**:1061-1075. DOI: 10.1007/s11357-012-9428-4

[82] Sumukadas D, Band M, Miller S, et al. Do ACE inhibitors improve the response to exercise training in functionally impaired older adults? A randomized controlled trial. The Journals of Gerontology Series A Biological Sciences and Medical Sciences. 2014;**69**:736-743. DOI: 10.1093/gerona/glt142

[83] Sumukadas D, Witham MD, Struthers AD, McMurdo ME. Effect of perindopril on physical function in elderly people with functional impairment: A randomized controlled trial. CMAJ: Canadian Medical Association Journal (Journal de l'Association medicale canadienne). 2007;**177**:867-874. DOI: 10.1503/cmaj.061339

[84] Murphy KT, Chee A, Trieu J, Naim T, Lynch GS. Inhibition of the renin-angiotensin system improves physiological outcomes in mice with mild or severe cancer cachexia. International Journal of Cancer. 2013;**133**:1234-1246. DOI: 10.1002/ijc.28128

[85] Fujita J, Mestre JR, Zeldis JB, Subbaramaiah K, Dannenberg AJ. Thalidomide and its analogues inhibit lipopolysaccharide-mediated induction of cyclooxygenase-2. Clinical Cancer Research: An Official Journal of the American Association for Cancer Research. 2001;**7**:3349-3355

[86] Kedar I, Mermershtain W, Ivgi H. Thalidomide reduces serum C-reactive protein and interleukin-6 and induces response to IL-2 in a fraction of metastatic renal cell cancer patients who failed IL-2-based therapy. International Journal of Cancer. 2004;**110**:260-265. DOI: 10.1002/ijc.20089

[87] Davis M, Lasheen W, Walsh D, Mahmoud F, Bicanovsky L, Lagman R. A phase II dose titration study of thalidomide for cancer-associated anorexia. Journal of Pain and Symptom Management. 2012;**43**:78-86. DOI: 10.1016/j.jpainsymman.2011.03.007

[88] Liu KH, Liao LM, Ro LS, Wu YL, Yeh TS. Thalidomide attenuates tumor growth and preserves fast-twitch skeletal muscle fibers in cholangiocarcinoma rats. Surgery. 2008;**143**:375-383. DOI: 10.1016/j.surg.2007.09.035

[89] Li TH, Lee PC, Lee KC, et al. Down-regulation of common NFκB-iNOS pathway by chronic thalidomide treatment improves hepatopulmonary syndrome and muscle wasting in rats with biliary cirrhosis. Scientific Reports. 2016;**6**:39405. DOI: 10.1038/srep39405

[90] Kaplan G, Thomas S, Fierer DS, et al. Thalidomide for the treatment of AIDS-associated wasting. AIDS Research and Human Retroviruses. 2000;**16**:1345-1355. DOI: 10.1089/08892220050140892

[91] Gordon JN, Trebble TM, Ellis RD, Duncan HD, Johns T, Goggin PM. Thalidomide in the treatment of cancer cachexia: A randomised placebo controlled trial. Gut. 2005;**54**:540-545. DOI: 10.1136/gut.2004.047563

[92] Wilkes EA, Selby AL, Cole AT, Freeman JG, Rennie MJ, Khan ZH. Poor tolerability of thalidomide in end-stage oesophageal cancer. European Journal of Cancer Care. 2011;**20**:593-600. DOI: 10.1111/j.1365-2354.2011.01255.x

[93] Tsujinaka T, Fujita J, Ebisui C, et al. Interleukin 6 receptor antibody inhibits muscle atrophy and modulates proteolytic systems in interleukin 6 transgenic mice. The Journal of Clinical Investigation. 1996;**97**:244-249. DOI: 10.1172/jci118398

[94] Narsale AA, Carson JA. Role of interleukin-6 in cachexia: Therapeutic implications. Current Opinion in Supportive and Palliative Care. 2014;**8**:321-327. DOI: 10.1097/spc.0000000000000091

[95] Bayliss TJ, Smith JT, Schuster M, Dragnev KH, Rigas JR. A humanized anti-IL-6 antibody (ALD518) in non-small cell lung cancer. Expert Opinion on Biological Therapy. 2011;**11**:1663-1668. DOI: 10.1517/14712598.2011.627850

[96] Jones SA, Scheller J, Rose-John S. Therapeutic strategies for the clinical blockade of IL-6/gp130 signaling. The Journal of Clinical Investigation. 2011;**121**:3375-3383. DOI: 10.1172/jci57158

[97] Song SN, Yoshizaki K. Tocilizumab for treating rheumatoid arthritis: An evaluation of pharmacokinetics/pharmacodynamics and clinical efficacy. Expert Opinion on Drug Metabolism & Toxicology. 2015;**11**:307-316. DOI: 10.1517/17425255.2015.992779

[98] Radigan KA, Nicholson TT, Welch LC, et al. Influenza A virus infection induces muscle wasting via IL-6 regulation of the E3 ubiquitin ligase atrogin-1. Journal of Immunology (Baltimore, Md.: 1950). 2019;**202**:484-493. DOI: 10.4049/jimmunol.1701433

[99] Yano T, Osanami A, Shimizu M, et al. Utility and safety of tocilizumab in Takayasu arteritis with severe heart failure and muscle wasting. ESC Heart Failure. 2019;**6**:894-897. DOI: 10.1002/ehf2.12487

[100] Bonetto A, Aydogdu T, Jin X, et al. JAK/STAT3 pathway inhibition blocks skeletal muscle wasting downstream of IL-6 and in experimental cancer cachexia. American Journal of Physiology. Endocrinology and Metabolism. 2012;**303**:E410-E421. DOI: 10.1152/ajpendo.00039.2012

[101] Zhang L, Pan J, Dong Y, et al. Stat3 activation links a C/EBPδ to myostatin pathway to stimulate loss of muscle mass. Cell Metabolism. 2013;**18**:368-379. DOI: 10.1016/j.cmet.2013.07.012

[102] Silva KA, Dong J, Dong Y, et al. Inhibition of Stat3 activation suppresses caspase-3 and the ubiquitin-proteasome system, leading to preservation of muscle mass in cancer cachexia. The Journal of Biological Chemistry. 2015;**290**:11177-11187. DOI: 10.1074/jbc.M115.641514

[103] Llovera M, Carbó N, García-Martínez C, et al. Anti-TNF treatment

reverts increased muscle ubiquitin gene expression in tumour-bearing rats. Biochemical and Biophysical Research Communications. 1996;**221**:653-655. DOI: 10.1006/bbrc.1996.0651

[104] Granado M, Martín AI, Priego T, López-Calderón A, Villanúa MA. Tumour necrosis factor blockade did not prevent the increase of muscular muscle RING finger-1 and muscle atrophy F-box in arthritic rats. The Journal of Endocrinology. 2006;**191**:319-326. DOI: 10.1677/joe.1.06931

[105] Wiedenmann B, Malfertheiner P, Friess H, et al. A multicenter, phase II study of infliximab plus gemcitabine in pancreatic cancer cachexia. The Journal of Supportive Oncology. 2008;**6**:18-25

[106] Subramaniam K, Fallon K, Ruut T, et al. Infliximab reverses inflammatory muscle wasting (sarcopenia) in Crohn's disease. Alimentary Pharmacology & Therapeutics. 2015;**41**:419-428. DOI: 10.1111/apt.13058

[107] DeBoer MD, Lee AM, Herbert K, et al. Increases in IGF-1 after anti-TNF-α therapy are associated with bone and muscle accrual in pediatric Crohn disease. The Journal of Clinical Endocrinology and Metabolism. 2018;**103**:936-945. DOI: 10.1210/jc.2017-01916

[108] Chen CY, Tsai CY, Lee PC, Lee SD. Long-term etanercept therapy favors weight gain and ameliorates cachexia in rheumatoid arthritis patients: Roles of gut hormones and leptin. Current Pharmaceutical Design. 2013;**19**:1956-1964. DOI: 10.2174/1381612811319100014

[109] Wu C, Fernandez SA, Criswell T, et al. Disrupting cytokine signaling in pancreatic cancer: A phase I/II study of etanercept in combination with gemcitabine in patients with advanced disease. Pancreas. 2013;**42**:813-818. DOI: 10.1097/MPA.0b013e318279b87f

[110] Hong DS, Hui D, Bruera E, et al. MABp1, a first-in-class true human antibody targeting interleukin-1α in refractory cancers: An open-label, phase 1 dose-escalation and expansion study. The Lancet Oncology. 2014;**15**:656-666. DOI: 10.1016/s1470-2045(14)70155-x

[111] Hickish T, Andre T, Wyrwicz L, et al. MABp1 as a novel antibody treatment for advanced colorectal cancer: A randomised, double-blind, placebo-controlled, phase 3 study. The Lancet Oncology. 2017;**18**:192-201. DOI: 10.1016/s1470-2045(17)30006-2

[112] Hong DS, Janku F, Naing A, et al. Xilonix, a novel true human antibody targeting the inflammatory cytokine interleukin-1 alpha, in non-small cell lung cancer. Investigational New Drugs. 2015;**33**:621-631. DOI: 10.1007/s10637-015-0226-6

[113] Kurzrock R, Hickish T, Wyrwicz L, et al. Interleukin-1 receptor antagonist levels predict favorable outcome after bermekimab, a first-in-class true human interleukin-1α antibody, in a phase III randomized study of advanced colorectal cancer. Oncoimmunology. 2019;**8**:1551651. DOI: 10.1080/2162402x.2018.1551651

[114] Yadava RS, Foff EP, Yu Q, et al. TWEAK/Fn14, a pathway and novel therapeutic target in myotonic dystrophy. Human Molecular Genetics. 2015;**24**:2035-2048. DOI: 10.1093/hmg/ddu617

[115] Bowerman M, Salsac C, Coque E, et al. Tweak regulates astrogliosis, microgliosis and skeletal muscle atrophy in a mouse model of amyotrophic lateral sclerosis. Human Molecular Genetics. 2015;**24**:3440-3456. DOI: 10.1093/hmg/ddv094

[116] Johnston AJ, Murphy KT, Jenkinson L, et al. Targeting of Fn14 prevents cancer-induced cachexia and prolongs survival.

Cell. 2015;**162**:1365-1378. DOI: 10.1016/j.cell.2015.08.031

[117] Zhou X, Wang JL, Lu J, et al. Reversal of cancer cachexia and muscle wasting by ActRIIB antagonism leads to prolonged survival. Cell. 2010;**142**:531-543. DOI: 10.1016/j.cell.2010.07.011

[118] Roth SM, Walsh S. Myostatin: A therapeutic target for skeletal muscle wasting. Current Opinion in Clinical Nutrition and Metabolic Care. 2004;**7**:259-263. DOI: 10.1097/00075197-200405000-00004

[119] Benny Klimek ME, Aydogdu T, Link MJ, Pons M, Koniaris LG, Zimmers TA. Acute inhibition of myostatin-family proteins preserves skeletal muscle in mouse models of cancer cachexia. Biochemical and Biophysical Research Communications. 2010;**391**:1548-1554. DOI: 10.1016/j.bbrc.2009.12.123

[120] Becker C, Lord SR, Studenski SA, et al. Myostatin antibody (LY2495655) in older weak fallers: A proof-of-concept, randomised, phase 2 trial. The Lancet Diabetes & Endocrinology. 2015;**3**:948-957. DOI: 10.1016/s2213-8587(15)00298-3

[121] Golan T, Geva R, Richards D, et al. LY2495655, an antimyostatin antibody, in pancreatic cancer: A randomized, phase 2 trial. Journal of Cachexia, Sarcopenia and Muscle. 2018;**9**:871-879. DOI: 10.1002/jcsm.12331

[122] Attie KM, Borgstein NG, Yang Y, et al. A single ascending-dose study of muscle regulator ACE-031 in healthy volunteers. Muscle & Nerve. 2013;**47**:416-423. DOI: 10.1002/mus.23539

[123] Campbell C, McMillan HJ, Mah JK, et al. Myostatin inhibitor ACE-031 treatment of ambulatory boys with Duchenne muscular dystrophy: Results of a randomized, placebo-controlled clinical trial. Muscle & Nerve. 2017;**55**:458-464. DOI: 10.1002/mus.25268

[124] Lach-Trifilieff E, Minetti GC, Sheppard K, et al. An antibody blocking activin type II receptors induces strong skeletal muscle hypertrophy and protects from atrophy. Molecular and Cellular Biology. 2014;**34**:606-618. DOI: 10.1128/mcb.01307-13

[125] Amato AA, Sivakumar K, Goyal N, et al. Treatment of sporadic inclusion body myositis with bimagrumab. Neurology. 2014;**83**:2239-2246. DOI: 10.1212/wnl.0000000000001070

[126] Rooks D, Praestgaard J, Hariry S, et al. Treatment of sarcopenia with bimagrumab: Results from a phase II, randomized, controlled, proof-of-concept study. Journal of the American Geriatrics Society. 2017;**65**:1988-1995. DOI: 10.1111/jgs.14927

[127] Polkey MI, Praestgaard J, Berwick A, et al. Activin type II receptor blockade for treatment of muscle depletion in chronic obstructive pulmonary disease. A randomized trial. American Journal of Respiratory and Critical Care Medicine. 2019;**199**:313-320. DOI: 10.1164/rccm.201802-0286OC

[128] Mori-Yoshimura M, Yamashita S, Suzuki N, et al. Late phase II/III study of BYM338 in patients with sporadic inclusion body myositis (RESILIENT): Japanese cohort data. Rinsho Shinkeigaku (Clinical Neurology). 2019;**59**:806-813. DOI: 10.5692/clinicalneurol.cn-001325

[129] Pascual López A, Roqué i Figuls M, Urrútia Cuchi G, et al. Systematic review of megestrol acetate in the treatment of anorexia-cachexia syndrome. Journal of Pain and Symptom Management. 2004;**27**:360-369. DOI: 10.1016/j.jpainsymman.2003.09.007

[130] McCarthy HD, Crowder RE, Dryden S, Williams G. Megestrol acetate stimulates food and water intake in the rat: Effects on regional hypothalamic neuropeptide Y concentrations. European Journal of Pharmacology. 1994;**265**:99-102. DOI: 10.1016/0014-2999(94)90229-1

[131] Mantovani G, Macciò A, Massa E, Madeddu C. Managing cancer-related anorexia/cachexia. Drugs. 2001;**61**:499-514. DOI: 10.2165/00003495-200161040-00004

[132] Ronga I, Gallucci F, Riccardi F, Uomo G. Anorexia-cachexia syndrome in pancreatic cancer: Recent advances and new pharmacological approach. Advances in Medical Sciences. 2014;**59**:1-6. DOI: 10.1016/j.advms.2013.11.001

[133] Wang J, Wang Y, Tong M, Pan H, Li D. New prospect for cancer cachexia: Medical cannabinoid. Journal of Cancer. 2019;**10**:716-720. DOI: 10.7150/jca.28246

[134] Brisbois TD, de Kock IH, Watanabe SM, et al. Delta-9-tetrahydrocannabinol may palliate altered chemosensory perception in cancer patients: Results of a randomized, double-blind, placebo-controlled pilot trial. Annals of Oncology: Official Journal of the European Society for Medical Oncology. 2011;**22**:2086-2093. DOI: 10.1093/annonc/mdq727

[135] Turcott JG, Del Rocío Guillen Núñez M, Flores-Estrada D, et al. The effect of nabilone on appetite, nutritional status, and quality of life in lung cancer patients: A randomized, double-blind clinical trial. Supportive Care in Cancer: Official Journal of the Multinational Association of Supportive Care in Cancer. 2018;**26**:3029-3038. DOI: 10.1007/s00520-018-4154-9

[136] Côté M, Trudel M, Wang C, Fortin A. Improving quality of life with nabilone during radiotherapy treatments for head and neck cancers: A randomized double-blind placebo-controlled trial. Annals of Otology, Rhinology, and Laryngology. 2016;**125**:317-324. DOI: 10.1177/0003489415612801

[137] Alamdari N, Aversa Z, Castillero E, et al. Resveratrol prevents dexamethasone-induced expression of the muscle atrophy-related ubiquitin ligases atrogin-1 and MuRF1 in cultured myotubes through a SIRT1-dependent mechanism. Biochemical and Biophysical Research Communications. 2012;**417**:528-533. DOI: 10.1016/j.bbrc.2011.11.154

[138] Wang DT, Yin Y, Yang YJ, et al. Resveratrol prevents TNF-α-induced muscle atrophy via regulation of Akt/mTOR/FoxO1 signaling in C2C12 myotubes. International Immunopharmacology. 2014;**19**:206-213. DOI: 10.1016/j.intimp.2014.02.002

[139] Momken I, Stevens L, Bergouignan A, et al. Resveratrol prevents the wasting disorders of mechanical unloading by acting as a physical exercise mimetic in the rat. FASEB Journal: Official Publication of the Federation of American Societies for Experimental Biology. 2011;**25**:3646-3660. DOI: 10.1096/fj.10-177295

[140] Chen X, Wu Y, Yang T, et al. Salidroside alleviates cachexia symptoms in mouse models of cancer cachexia via activating mTOR signalling. Journal of Cachexia, Sarcopenia and Muscle. 2016;7:225-232. DOI: 10.1002/jcsm.12054

[141] Chen L, Chen L, Wan L, et al. Matrine improves skeletal muscle atrophy by inhibiting E3 ubiquitin ligases and activating the Akt/mTOR/FoxO3α signaling pathway in C2C12

myotubes and mice. Oncology Reports. 2019;**42**:479-494. DOI: 10.3892/or.2019.7205

[142] Chen L, Xu W, Yang Q, et al. Imperatorin alleviates cancer cachexia and prevents muscle wasting via directly inhibiting STAT3. Pharmacological Research. 2020;**158**:104871. DOI: 10.1016/j.phrs.2020.104871

[143] Yang Q, Wan L, Zhou Z, et al. Parthenolide from *Parthenium integrifolium* reduces tumor burden and alleviate cachexia symptoms in the murine CT-26 model of colorectal carcinoma. Phytomedicine: International Journal of Phytotherapy and Phytopharmacology. 2013;**20**:992-998. DOI: 10.1016/j.phymed.2013.04.020

[144] Yu R, Chen JA, Xu J, et al. Suppression of muscle wasting by the plant-derived compound ursolic acid in a model of chronic kidney disease. Journal of Cachexia, Sarcopenia and Muscle. 2017;**8**:327-341. DOI: 10.1002/jcsm.12162

[145] Chen L, Yang Q, Zhang H, et al. Cryptotanshinone prevents muscle wasting in CT26-induced cancer cachexia through inhibiting STAT3 signaling pathway. Journal of Ethnopharmacology. 2020;**260**:113066. DOI: 10.1016/j.jep.2020.113066

Chapter 6

Nutritional Approaches for Attenuating Muscle Atrophy

Muneshige Shimizu and Kunihiro Sakuma

Abstract

Muscle atrophy occurs under a number of different conditions, including disuse and aging accompanied by the onset of sarcopenia. Although muscle mass is reduced by decreased protein synthesis and/or increased protein degradation, the mechanisms of disuse muscle atrophy and sarcopenia differ. Therefore, nutrition strategies need to be customized for each type of muscle atrophy. Difficulties are associated with assessing the efficacy of nutrients for preventing sarcopenia due to uncontrolled factors in human studies. We herein (a) summarize nutritional epidemiology evidence related to sarcopenia from recent systematic reviews, (b) review nutrient supplementation for attenuating sarcopenia through dietary control, and (c) provide evidence for the efficacy of nutrient supplementation for treating disuse muscle atrophy under dietary control. Epidemiological studies have indicated that diets with a sufficient intake of beneficial foods are useful for preventing sarcopenia. Supplementation with vitamin D and leucine-enriched whey protein have been suggested to help attenuate sarcopenia in geriatric patients, particularly those who are unable to exercise. Further studies are needed to clarify the effects of protein and amino acid supplementation on muscle mass and strength. High-quality studies with controlled diets and physical activities are required to clarify the effects of nutritional interventions on both types of muscle atrophy.

Keywords: diet quality, muscle atrophy, disuse, sarcopenia, epidemiology

1. Introduction

Muscle mass and strength have been linked to overall health and mortality [1, 2], and improvements in skeletal muscle properties and the prevention of muscle wasting with disuse/atrophy are essential for all individuals, particularly inactive older adults [3]. Sarcopenia is characterized by the loss of skeletal muscle mass and physical function (muscle strength or physical performance) with advancing age [4–6]. It is associated with physical disability, poor quality of life, and increased mortality in older adults [5]. Although the loss of muscle mass and physical function is associated with aging, rates of decline vary across the population [7]. Therefore, modifiable behavioral factors, such as diet, may influence the development of sarcopenia. Since a poor diet and nutritional status are common among the elderly [8–10], improvements in these factors may contribute to the prevention and treatment of sarcopenia, thereby promoting better health in later life for this population [11].

The term *diet quality* describes how well an individual's diet conforms to dietary recommendations using a principal component or factor analysis [12, 13]. In older adults, a higher quality diet leads to several positive health outcomes, including a reduced risk of common age-related diseases and greater longevity. For example, a high quality diet is associated with a significantly reduced risk of all-cause mortality, cardiovascular disease, cancer, type 2 diabetes, and neurodegenerative disease, as well as reduced mortality in cancer survivors [14–17].

While there is growing evidence linking healthier diets with greater muscle strength and better physical performance outcomes in older adults, limited information is currently available on how diet quality influences sarcopenia in older adults [11, 18]. A recent systematic review concluded that the number of longitudinal studies was too small to reach concrete conclusions; however, there is growing evidence for the benefits of adhering to a Mediterranean diet [19–21]. The next section summarizes current epidemiological evidence for the relationship between diet quality and sarcopenia in older adults.

2. Nutritional approaches for attenuating muscle atrophy

2.1 Nutritional epidemiology evidence related to sarcopenia

The world's population is getting older [22]. Based on a 2017 report, the number of adults aged 60 years and older will increase worldwide, from 962 million (or one in eight individuals) in 2017 to 2.1 billion (one in five) by the middle of the 21st century [23]. Several environmental and lifestyle factors may modify the aging process [24], including physical activity [25, 26] and diet [27–29].

A large number of observational and intervention studies have used a single-nutrient approach to investigate the relationship between diet and muscle health in aging. However, difficulties are associated with isolating the influence of one dietary component on health outcomes from other components as well as obtaining a clearer understanding of how dietary components interact within a whole diet to affect health outcomes. Previous studies using a whole-diet approach were conducted to clarify the role diet quality plays in muscle health with aging [30–33].

Two main methods of defining diet quality—*a priori* (hypothesis-driven) and *a posteriori* (data driven)—have been used to investigate the relationships between diet quality and muscle health in epidemiological studies on muscle aging. The *a priori* method defines diet quality as adherence to predefined dietary scores or indices based on current knowledge on what constitutes a healthy diet for a particular health condition (e.g., cardiovascular disease or diabetes). In this method, higher scores reflect the greater consumption of beneficial foods (e.g., fruits, vegetables, lean meat, fish, nuts, and low-fat foods) and lower consumption of nutrient-poor foods (e.g., sweets, processed meat, refined grains, and trans-fats) [34–36]. In contrast, the *a posteriori* method is exploratory, using all available dietary data to define diet quality. This method may be used to describe a population's normal diet, which may or may not be related to particular health outcomes. In this method, multivariate statistical tools (e.g., a factor principal component analysis [PCA] and cluster analysis) may be used to assess diet quality. While these two tools follow markedly different procedures, they may be used in tandem to improve the interpretability of the data obtained from each method [37].

We reviewed nutritional epidemiology studies on the role of diet quality in muscle health and function in older adults (**Table 1**). Only eight studies reported a relationship between diet quality (i.e., the amount of nutrients consumed and/or the uptake of specific nutrients from foods) and sarcopenia components [38–45]. Five of these studies were cross-sectional, while three were longitudinal. Study sample sizes ranged between 156 and 2983 participants. The majority of studies

Reference	Population	Study design	Diet quality (DQ)	Physical function
Robinson et al. (2008) [38]	n = 2983 community-dwelling men (n = 1569) and women (n = 1414), 65.7 ± 2.9 years (men) 66.6 ± 2.7 years (women)	Cross-sectional	Administered FFQ based on EPIC Questionnaire 18, pertaining to the 3-month period preceding the interview.	Men and women with high prudent diet scores had stronger grip strengths.
Martin et al. (2011) [39]	n = 628 community-dwelling men (n = 348) and women (n = 280), 67.8 ± 2.5 years (men) 68.1 ± 2.5 years (women)	Cross-sectional	Administered FFQ pertaining to the 3-month period preceding the interview Data-driven: PCA. A "prudent" dietary pattern was identified.	In women, a higher prudent diet score was associated with a shorter 3-m walk time, shorter chair-rise time, and better balance.
Bollwein et al. (2013) [40]	n = 192 community-dwelling men and women, 83 ± 4 years	Cross-sectional	Administered FFQ of the German part of the EPIC study. Dietary indices: Adherence to a Mediterranean dietary pattern was assessed using the MED score	A relationship was observed between a high MED score and lower risk of a slow walking speed.
Rahi et al. (2014) [41]	n = 156 community-dwelling men (n = 94) and women (n = 62) with type 2 diabetes, 74.3 ± 4.2 years (men) 75.0 ± 4.2 years (women)	Longitudinal	Three non-consecutive 24-h dietary recalls. Dietary indices; DQ was evaluated at recruitment using the Canadian Healthy Eating Index (C-HEI).	Good DQ was combined with stable or increased physical activity, and muscle strength losses were minimal in diabetic older males.
Hashemi et al. (2015) [42]	n = 300 elderly men and women (55 years old and older), 66.8 ± 7.2 years	Cross-sectional	Three major dietary patterns (DP) were identified. a. DP1, Mediterranean b. DP2, Western c. DP3, Mixed	Participants in the highest tertile of DP1 had a lower odds ratio for sarcopenia than those in the lowest tertile.

Reference	Population	Study design	Diet quality (DQ)	Physical function
Granic et al. (2016) [43]	n = 791 men (n = 302) and women (n = 489), living either at home or in a care facility, 68.7 ± 0.3 years	Longitudinal	Three dietary patterns were identified. a. DP1, High Red Meat b. DP2, Low Meat c. DP3, High Butter	Men in DP1 had worse overall hand grip strength and slower timed up and go than those in DP2. Women in DP3 had slower timed up and go than those in DP2. Men in DP3 had a steeper decline in hand grip strength than those in DP1.
Perälä et al. (2016) [44]	n = 1072 participants, elderly men and women, 61.3 ± 0.2 years	Longitudinal	Dietary indices: The *a priori*-defined Nordic diet score (NDS) was calculated as a measure of a healthy Nordic diet.	Women in the highest fourth of the NDS had a 5-point higher Senior Fitness Test score on average than those in the lowest fourth.
Suthutvoravut et al. (2020) [45]	n = 1241 community-dwelling men (n = 646) and women (n = 595), 74.6 ± 5.5 years	Cross-sectional	Three dietary patterns were identified. a. DP1, high factor loading for fish, tofu, vegetables, and fruits b DP2, high factor loading for fish, rice, and miso soup c. DP3, high factor loading for noodles	Men with the lowest tertile of the DP1 score had a higher likelihood of being sarcopenic. Women with the lowest tertile of the DP2 score had a moderate likelihood of being sarcopenic.

Table 1.
Summary of diet quality and physical function in older adults.

were conducted in a community setting (e.g., a nursing home or care facility) and with participants whose mean age ranged between 65 and 75 years.

Robinson et al. examined the relationship between diet quality and grip strength in older men and women [38]. A food frequency questionnaire (FFQ) based on the European Prospective Investigation of Cancer (EPIC) questionnaire was used to assess the subject's diet. They used the FFQ that contained 129 foods and food groups and assessed the average frequency of the consumption of the listed foods over the three months preceding the interview. Nutrient intake for each food item consumed was calculated by multiplying the nutrient content listed in the UK national food composition database or manufacturer composition data. The 129 foods listed in the FFQ were divided into 54 food groups based on similarity and nutrient compositions. The PCA of the reported weekly consumption frequencies of these food groups was used to define diet patterns. The *prudent* diet was characterized by the high consumption of fruit, vegetables, whole grain cereals, and fatty fish and by the low consumption of white bread, chips, sugar, and full-fat dairy products. Participants with higher prudent diet scores had stronger grip strengths. In addition, an increase was observed in grip strength of 0.43 kg in men and 0.48 kg in women for each additional fatty fish portion consumed per week.

Martin et al. investigated the relationship between diet and physical performance (measured using a short physical performance battery) in a group of men and women living in West Hertfordshire who were part of the Hertfordshire Cohort Study [39]. Nutrient intake for each food item consumed was calculated by multiplying the nutrient content listed in the UK national food composition database or manufacturer composition data. Higher prudent diet scores were related to shorter three-meter walk times and shorter chair-rise times in women. Additionally, inverse relationships were observed between physical function and the consumption of vegetables, whitefish, shellfish, and oily fish. These findings indicate that a relationship exists between diet variations in community-dwelling older women and differences in physical performance. However, further studies are needed to clarify the role of diet variations in physical performance, particularly in men.

Bollwein et al. examined whether the risk of frailty was significantly reduced in participants who scored in the highest quartile for Mediterranean diet consumption (MED) [40]. This scoring is an alternative to the MED scoring used by Fung et al. [46], who adapted the original MED score used by Trichopoulou et al. [47] for a non-Mediterranean population. They combined FFQ foods into nine nutritional characteristics, classified as either beneficial (vegetables, legumes, fruits, unrefined cereals, nuts, fish, high monounsaturated fatty acid [MUFA]/saturated fatty acid [SFA] foods, and moderate alcohol consumption) or detrimental (red and processed meats) to health, to calculate the score, and found an inverse correlation between a low walking speed and MED scores. Moreover, a relationship was observed between high diet quality (high MED score) and slow walking speed in older men and women.

Rahi et al. investigated the relationship between diet quality and muscle strength changes over three years in diabetic participants aged 67 to 84 years [41]. Diet quality was evaluated at recruitment using the validated Diet Quality Index-Canada and nine-item Canadian Healthy Eating Index (C-HEI) [48]. Diet quality was calculated using data from the mean of three, non-consecutive, 24-hour dietary recalls collected using the five-step, multiple-pass method [49]. The C-HEI has nine components. The first four components evaluate the extent to which respondents meet age and gender-based recommendations for the number of portions eaten from each of the four groups of Canada's Food Guide (grain products, vegetables and fruits, milk and alternatives, and meat and alternatives). The next four items reflect Canadian nutritional recommendations for moderation: the daily percentage of energy from total fat, the daily percentage of energy from saturated fat, cholesterol intake (mg), and sodium intake (mg). The final component, dietary variety (adapted from the Dietary Diversity Score), was assessed as the daily consumption of at least one food from each food group. The findings obtained indicated that the combination of a high diet quality with stable or increased physical activity minimized muscle strength losses in diabetic older males over the three-year follow-up period.

Hashemi et al. investigated whether adherence to a particular dietary pattern was associated with sarcopenia among elderly adults in a district of Teheran, Iran [42]. A semiquantitative FFQ was used to survey the dietary intake of 300 randomly-selected older men and women. They evaluated the dietary patterns of participants using PCA. Participants in the highest tertile of the Mediterranean dietary pattern had a lower odds ratio for developing sarcopenia than those in the lowest tertile. In contrast, adherence to the Western dietary pattern (characterized by the high consumption of sugar, soy, and fast foods) and mixed dietary pattern (characterized by the high consumption of animal proteins, potatoes, and refined grains) did not affect the odds of developing sarcopenia. These findings suggested that Mediterranean diet adherence was associated with a lower odds ratio for the development of sarcopenia among older Iranian individuals.

Granic et al. examined the relationship between previously established dietary patterns and declines in muscle strength and physical performance among older adults [43]. In total, 791 participants were followed for five years to detect changes in grip strength and timed up and go test (TUG) scores. Trained research nurses kept a detailed record of food intake on the previous day for each participant on two different days of the week, at least one week apart. Each food had a unique food code (>2000), and intakes were entered into a Microsoft Access-based dietary data system, then further grouped into 118 food groups based on McCance and Widdowson's composition of foods [50, 51]. These 118 groups were combined into 33 food groups based on food/nutrient composition similarities and then classified as either absent or present in each participant's food intake. Participants were divided into three groups: dietary pattern 1 (DP1; high red meat); dietary pattern 2 (DP2; low meat); and dietary pattern 3 (DP3; high butter). The findings obtained showed that men in DP1 had worse overall grip strength, whereas those in DP3 had steeper grip strength declines than those in DP2. Additionally, TUG scores were significantly longer for men in DP1 and women in DP3 than those in DP2. Therefore, diets high in red meats, potatoes, gravy, and butter appear to adversely affect muscle strength and physical performance in later life.

Perälä et al. researched whether the consumption of a healthy Nordic diet for 10 years was associated with improved physical performance measures [44]. After the diets of 1072 participants (mean age 67 years) had been examined using a validated 128-item FFQ, the *a priori* Nordic diet score was calculated. The diet items checked included Nordic fruits and berries, vegetables, cereals, low-fat milk, fish, red and processed meat, alcohol, polyunsaturated omega-3 fatty acids (PUFA)/SFA and trans-fatty acids ratios, and total fat. Since participants had a mean age of 71 years, their physical performance was measured using the Senior Fitness Test (SFT), and an overall SFT score was calculated. The findings obtained revealed that women with the highest diet scores had 17% better in that of walk, 16% better in that of arm curl, and 20% better in that of chair-stand than women with the lowest diet scores. These findings indicated that women who consumed a healthy Nordic diet had better physical performance (i.e., better aerobic endurance and upper and lower body strength) 10 years later.

Suthutvoravut et al. investigated the relationship between dietary patterns and sarcopenia in a sample of older community-dwelling Japanese adults [45]. The sample included 1241 older adults aged 65 years and older who were not eligible for long-term care. Dietary intake by participants was assessed using the brief self-administered diet history questionnaire. Dietary patterns were identified using both PCA and Japanese diet scores (soybeans and soybean products, fish, vegetables, pickles, mushrooms, seaweeds, and fruits). Participants were classified into three groups: dietary pattern 1 (DP1; high factor loading for the consumption of fish, tofu, vegetables, and fruits found in typical Japanese side dishes); dietary pattern 2 (DP2; high factor loading for fish, rice, and miso soup found in typical Japanese main dishes); and dietary pattern 3 (DP3; high factor loading for noodles). The findings obtained showed that men with the lowest tertile DP1 score had a higher likelihood of being sarcopenic, while women with the lowest tertile DP2 score had a moderate likelihood of being sarcopenic. Additionally, low adherence to Japanese dietary patterns increased with the prevalence of sarcopenia in both genders.

Many traditional regional diets may have similar benefits to those described here. We then focused on diets with demonstrated effects on muscle mass, reported by randomized controlled trials that investigated diet quality using precise parameters. For example, the traditional diets of Korea and China may be beneficial for preventing sarcopenia in the populations of these countries. Healthier diets are higher in plant-based food and lower in animal-based foods than Western diets. Further epidemiological studies are needed to investigate the relationship between healthy diets and development of sarcopenia throughout the world, particularly in developing countries.

2.2 Nutrient supplementation for attenuating sarcopenia

Skeletal muscle is a dynamic, plastic tissue with a mass that is regulated by the balance between the rates of muscle protein synthesis and breakdown. Adopting an appropriate dietary strategy is crucial for facilitating an anabolic response that may prevent muscle wasting with atrophy by suppressing the breakdown of muscle protein. An adequate nutrient intake is essential for maintaining and improving muscle properties. Many supplements have been proposed to enhance muscle mass and strength. More than 50% of adults in the United States take some form of dietary supplement to improve their health or well-being [52]. However, there is no scientific evidence for the effectiveness of many of these supplements. In some cases, their use has been linked to serious adverse side effects. This section summarizes the effects of several popular nutritional supplements when administered under strict dietary controls, either alone or in combination with other supplements.

In a randomized study, Tieland et al. examined the effects of 24 weeks of dietary protein supplementation on muscle mass, strength, and physical performance in a sample of frail older adults [53]. This study included 65 frail participants who were allocated to either the daily protein supplementation group (15 g protein consumed at breakfast and lunch) or placebo group (0 g protein at breakfast and lunch). Participants recorded their food intake for three days with the help of trained dieticians. Dietary intake data were coded (the type of food, time of intake, and amount), and energy and macronutrient intakes were calculated using a food-calculation system from the 2006 Dutch food composition database. The findings obtained indicated that skeletal muscle mass did not change in either the protein or placebo group following the 24-week intervention. However, leg extension strength increased more in the protein group than in the placebo group. Furthermore, physical performance significantly improved (from 8.9 to 10.0 points) in the protein group, but not in the placebo group. Therefore, while dietary protein supplementation appeared to improve physical performance in frail older adults, it did not increase their skeletal muscle mass.

Kim et al. investigated whether protein-energy supplementation prevented functional declines in frail older adults with a low socioeconomic status [54]. In that study, 84 frail elderly participants were assigned to either an intervention or control group. The intervention group received two 200-ml cans of commercial liquid formula (an additional 400 kcal of energy, 25 g of protein, 9.4 g of essential amino acids, and 400 ml of water) each day for 12 weeks, while the control group did not. Dietary intake was assessed in three, non-consecutive 24-hour recall sessions (one face-to-face and two by telephone; weekday and weekend ratio of 2:1) to show the nutritional status. The same research dietitian coded dietary data, and a nutrient analysis was performed using CAN-Pro 3.0. No significant changes were observed in grip strength in either group; however, physical functioning, usual gait speed, and TUG scores were significantly better in the protein group than in the control group. Therefore, protein-energy supplementation administered to frail older adults with a low socioeconomic status appeared to reduce the progression of functional decline.

Veronese et al. investigated whether 12 weeks of oral magnesium supplementation improved physical performance in healthy older women [55]. In that study, 124 participants were grouped into either a treatment group (300 mg of magnesium/day) or control group (no treatment). A dietary assessment was examined by a modified method including an estimated three-day record and a questionnaire about the frequency that participants generally ate certain foods. They used the data from the previous month as a reference and calculated the macronutrients and micronutrients of usual food intake by a national food composition table. After 12 weeks of supplementation with magnesium, the treatment group had significantly higher total short physical performance battery scores, chair-stand times, and four-minute walking speeds than the control group. These findings indicated that magnesium supplementation prevented or delayed age-related physical performance declines.

Roma et al. examined the effects of PUFA supplementation on the parameters of body composition, muscle strength, and physical performance in the elderly [56]. Fifty participants were randomly assigned to a PUFA-treated group (receiving 1.3 g of PUFA and 10 mg of vitamin E) or control group (receiving 11 mg of vitamin E). Participants were assessed using the mini nutritional assessment (composed of six questions related to decreased food intake in the three months before the test) and a 12-question survey on diet (number of meals consumed and consumption of protein, fruits, vegetables, and liquids) and the ability to feed themselves. No significant between-group differences were observed in muscle mass, grip strength, or TUG scores. Therefore, the 12-week PUFA supplementation did not appear to affect the parameters evaluated in elderly individuals with a decreased muscle mass.

Bauer et al. sought to test the hypothesis that a specific oral nutritional supplement may improve selected sarcopenia measures [57]. The active group (n = 184) consumed a vitamin D and leucine-enriched whey protein nutritional supplement twice daily for 13 weeks. The control group (n = 196) consumed an iso-caloric control product twice daily for 13 weeks. A dietary assessment was completed at baseline and week 13 using three-day prospective diet records for two weekdays and one weekend day. Additional energy and protein intakes from both supplements were added to habitual three-day intakes to assess total intake. The active group gained more appendicular muscle mass and performed better in the chair-stand test than the control group. These findings demonstrated that specific nutritional supplementation alone may benefit geriatric patients, particularly those unable to exercise.

Porter et al. investigated whether participants following an enhanced protein regimen have greater functional status improvements and better lean muscle mass preservation than control group participants [58]. In that study, 67 obese older adults were randomly assigned to either a traditional weight loss regimen (control group) or one with a higher protein intake at each meal (protein group). Control group participants were prescribed a 500-kcal deficit diet (15% protein, 30% fat, and 55% carbohydrate), which met the recommended dietary allowance (RDA) for protein intake (0.8 g/kg of body weight). Protein group participants were also prescribed a 500-kcal deficit, but with a macronutrient distribution of 30% protein, 30% fat, and 40% carbohydrate, for a total prescribed protein intake of 1.2 g/kg. Both groups exhibited significant weight loss at the six-month endpoint. However, while both groups had improved muscle function, the Short Physical Performance Battery response was greater in the protein group than in the control group. These findings indicated that functionally limited obese adults undergoing a six-month weight loss intervention that included a meal-based protein enhancement lost similar amounts of weight, but had better functional improvements than the control group.

Only one of the studies used an iso-caloric control supplement to investigate the efficacy of a vitamin D and leucine-enriched whey protein nutritional supplement (not combined with exercise) for attenuating sarcopenia. To produce the most useful data, future studies that investigate whether a simple nutrient supplement contributes to the prevention of sarcopenia will need to use dietary control in a sample of more than 100 elderly participants. Evidence from two *in vivo* studies showed that calorie restriction or fasting may help to prevent reductions in muscle mass or strength [59, 60]. Future human studies need to focus on the effects of the removal of some nutrients from the diet, instead of solely assessing the effects of their addition, in order to obtain more useful data (**Table 2**).

2.3 Nutrient supplementation effects on muscle mass and strength during muscle disuse

A number of conditions, such as recovery from injury or illness or space flight, require prolonged periods of muscle disuse (i.e., unloading) in otherwise healthy individuals, resulting in the progressive loss of skeletal muscle mass that impairs functional strength, reduces the basal metabolic rate, and increases body fat mass. Therefore, prolonged muscle disuse is a significant health concern, particularly in aging populations. While nutrition is an important factor regulating muscle mass, the development of effective nutritional strategies that attenuate muscle loss during periods of muscle disuse warrants further efforts. **Table 3** shows an overview of studies that have assessed the efficacy of nutritional interventions for attenuating muscle disuse atrophy under controlled diet quality.

Paddon-Jones et al. examined whether supplementation with essential amino acids and carbohydrates offset the catabolic response to 28 days of bed rest [61]. Thirteen healthy male participants were randomly assigned to either the experimental or control groups. The control group consumed nutritionally mixed meals three times a day. The experimental group consumed the same meals plus 30 g of carbohydrate and 16.5 g of essential amino acids three times a day. The Harris-Benedict equation was used to estimate daily caloric requirements, according to the following formula: daily energy requirement (kcal) = $[66 + (13.7 \times kg) + (5 \times cm) - (6.8 \times yr)] \times 1.3$ (activity factor for bed rest). Participants were placed on a three-day rotating diet with daily nutrient intake evenly distributed between the three meals. The findings obtained revealed that the experimental group maintained lean leg mass throughout bed rest (+0.2 kg), whereas the control group lost mass (−0.4 kg). In addition, strength loss was more pronounced in the control group (exp group, −8.8 kg; cont group, −17.8 kg). Therefore, supplementation with essential amino acids and carbohydrates during bed rest appeared to provide an anabolic stimulus that ameliorated lean muscle mass loss in an otherwise catabolic environment. However, it currently remains unclear whether additional energy intake contributed to these findings.

Reference	Population	Diets	Nutritional intervention	Changes in muscle mass and strength	Physical function
Tieland et al. (2012) [53]	n = 65 frail elderly subjects	1935 kcal/day, 49% CHO, 35% fat, 16% protein (1.0 g protein/kg/day)	15 g protein × twice/day for 24 wks vs. non protein × twice/day for 24 wks	No change in muscle mass in both groups Significant increase in muscle strength in both groups.	Significantly improved physical performance in the protein group, but not in the control group
Kim et al. (2013) [54]	n = 84 frail elderly subjects, 78.7 ± 5.8 years	896 kcal/day (0.7 g protein/kg/day)	400 kcal (25 g protein, 9.4 g amino acids, 56 g carbohydrate, 9 g lipids, micronutrients)/day for 12 wks vs. non-supplemental control	No change in hand grip strength in both groups	Significantly improved physical functioning, usual gait speed, and timed up-and-go in the protein group, but not in the control group
Veronese et al. (2014) [55]	n = 124 elderly women, 71.5 ± 5.2 years	1490 kcal/day (383 mg magnesium/day)	300 mg magnesium/day for 12 wks vs. non-supplemental control	No change in hand grip strength in both groups	Significantly improved Short Physical Performance Battery score, chair-stand times, and 4-m walking speeds in the magnesium group, but not in the control group
Roma et al. (2015) [56]	n = 50 elderly subjects, 74.9 ± 7.9 years	Mini Nutritional Assessment score 24.1 ± 3.1 points	1.3 g omega-3 fatty acids/day for 12 wks vs. non-supplemental control	No differences in muscle mass or hand grip in both groups	No differences in timed up-and-go in both groups
Bauer et al. (2015) [57]	n = 380 sarcopenic primarily independent-living older adults, 77.7 ± 6.9 years	1612 kcal/day (1.0 g protein/kg/day)	800 IU vitamin D + 20 g whey protein +3 g leucine twice/day for 13 wks (active) vs. iso-caloric control	Significantly higher appendicular muscle mass in the active group than in the control	Significantly improved chair-stand test in the active group from those in the control group
Porter et al. (2016) [58]	n = 67 obese older adults with a Short Physical Performance Battery (SPPB) score of 4–10, 68.2 ± 5.6 years	1458 kcal/day, 55% CHO, 30% fat, 15% protein (0.8 g protein/kg/day)	30 g protein × 3 times/day for 6 mo vs. non-supplemental control	No differences in lean body mass or hand grip in both groups	Significantly improved total and chair-stand scores in the protein group from those in the control group

Table 2.
Summary of effects of nutrient supplementation for attenuating sarcopenia.

Reference	Population	Diets	Nutritional intervention	Changes in muscle mass	Loss of strength
Paddon-Jones et al. (2004) [61]	n=13 young males, Bed rest (28 days)	2487 kcal/day, 59% CHO, 27% fat, 14% protein (1.0 g protein/kg/day)	30 g carbohydrate +16.5 g EAA vs. non-supplemental control	Leg lean mass maintained in EAA, but lost in the control	Significantly lower decrease of 11% in EAA than in the control (23% down)
Trappe et al. (2007) [62]	n = 24 young women, Bed rest (60 days)	1557 kcal/day, 56% CHO, 30% fat, 14% protein (1.0 g protein/kg/day)	1.0 (low), 1.6 (high) g/kg body mass/day dietary protein	Greater loss of quadriceps femoris muscle volume in high protein (24%) vs. low protein (21%)	19 ~ 33% decreased for the supine square in both groups
Ferrando et al. (2010) [63]	n = 21 elderly, Bed rest (10 days)	(0.8 g protein/kg/day)	15 g × 3 times/day EAA vs. the non-supplemental control	~6% decrease in leg lean mass in both groups	Better functional capacity in EAA than in control
Deutz et al. (2013) [64]	n=19 older adults, Bed rest (10 days)	1900 kcal/day (0.8 g protein/kg/day)	3 g/day HMB vs. non-supplemental control, 5 days prior to bed rest	Leg lean mass maintained in HMB, but lost in control	No difference in the knee extensor in both groups
Dirks et al. (2014) [65]	n = 23 elderly men, One-legged immobilization (5 days)	2150 kcal/day, 51% CHO, 33% fat, 16% protein (1.1 g protein/kg/day)	9.3 g carbohydrate +20.7 g protein +3.0 g fat twice/day vs. the non supplemental control	1.5 ~ 2.0% decrease in quadriceps CSA in both groups	8.3 ~ 9.3% decrease in maximal muscle strength in both groups
English et al. (2016) [66]	n=19 middle-aged adults, Bed rest (10 days)	2111 kcal/day, 55% CHO, 30% fat, 15% protein (1.1 g protein/kg/day)	4.5 g × 3 times/day leucine vs. 4.5 g × 3 times/day alanine	5.3 ~ 6.9% reduction in leg lean mass in both groups	Significantly smaller decrease of 7% in leucine than in alanine (15% down) with knee extensor peak torque
Holloway et al. (2019) [67]	n = 20 young men, One-legged immobilization (8 days)	2521 kcal/day (1.0 g protein/kg/day)	23.7 g × 3 times/day amino acids vs. 23.7 g × 3 times/day maltodextrin (iso-caloric control)	Significantly lower decrease of 3.1% in amino acids than in control (2.4% down) in quadriceps muscle volume	No difference in both groups in peak leg isometric torque

Table 3.
Summary of effects of nutritional interventions on muscle mass and strength during a period of muscle disuse.

Trappe et al. investigated whether nutritional countermeasures, consisting of additional protein and free leucine, reduced volume and strength losses in lower-limb skeletal muscle during 60 days of simulated weightlessness [62]. Young women were assigned to either the bed rest group (control) or the bedrest plus a nutrition countermeasure group (intervention). Dietary staff prepared all meals for both groups. These meals contained controlled amounts of total energy and macronutrients. The findings obtained demonstrated that thigh muscle (quadriceps femoris) volume decreased in both the control (−21%) and intervention groups (−24%). Moreover, both groups exhibited similar large decreases in isometric and dynamic (centric force, eccentric force, power, and work) muscle strength for the supine squat (−19% to −33%). Therefore, the nutrition countermeasure did not appear to be effective at offsetting volume or strength losses in lower-limb muscles. Furthermore, exercise countermeasures may need to be modified to protect the calf muscles of participants.

Ferrando et al. examined the effects of an increasing protein intake (through essential amino acid supplementation) in older individuals subjected to 10 days of bed rest on their lean body mass and muscle function [63]. Participants received either a placebo or 15 g of essential amino acids, three times a day throughout 10 days of bed rest. The placebo was a non-caloric diet soda. During diet stabilization and bed rest, subjects consumed a lacto-ovo vegetarian diet providing the RDA for protein (0.8 g/kg of protein per day). The diet consisted of a three-day rotation based on the Harris-Benedict equation designed to maintain body weight throughout the study. An activity factor of 1.3 was used to estimate daily energy requirements during bed rest. The findings obtained indicated that essential amino acids did not affect the maintenance of total or leg lean muscle mass. However, stair ascent power and standing plantar flexion appeared to be maintained with essential amino acid supplementation. Therefore, increasing protein intake above the RDA may preserve muscle function in elderly individuals during compulsory inactivity. However, this protocol may need to be operated under iso-caloric nutritional interventions.

Deutz et al. attempted to clarify whether beta-hydroxy-beta-methylbutyrate (HMB), a leucine metabolite, was capable of attenuating muscle decline in healthy older adults during 10 days of bed rest [64]. Healthy older adults were randomly assigned to a control group or HMB group (Ca-HMB, 1.5 g twice daily, total 3 g/day). Participants were fed a metabolically controlled diet for diet stabilization, providing the RDA for protein intake (0.8 g protein/kg of body weight per day). Total calorie needs were estimated using the Harris–Benedict equation for resting energy expenditure. An activity factor of 1.35 was used to estimate daily energy requirements during bedrest. The study protocol significantly decreased total lean body mass in the control group. In contrast, the treatment with HMB prevented these declines in all but one participant in the HMB group. However, differences in functional parameters were not observed between the two groups. These findings indicated that HMB supplementation contributed to the preservation of muscle mass during 10 days of bed rest. Further studies using larger samples and iso-calorie conditions for nutritional interventions are needed to clarify the preventative effects of HMB on the acute decline in muscle mass.

Dirks et al. investigated whether protein supplementation preserved muscle mass during a short period of limb immobilization [65]. Healthy older men were subjected to five days of one-legged knee immobilization using a full-leg cast with or without the twice-daily administration of a dietary protein supplement (20.7 g of protein, 9.3 g of carbohydrate, and 3.0 g of fat). Weighted dietary intake records were completed by participants for the five-day immobilization period and on a separate consecutive five-day occasion, either before or after the immobilization period. Immobilization decreased the quadricep cross-sectional area by 1.5 and 2.0%, and muscle strength by 8.3 and 9.3% in the control and protein groups, respectively. These findings indicated that dietary protein supplementation (~20 g twice daily) did not attenuate muscle loss during short-term muscle disuse in healthy older men.

English et al. investigated whether leucine protects skeletal muscle health during bed rest [66]. In that study, a group of middle-aged adults were randomly assigned to a leucine group (4.5 g leucine × 3 times/day) or alanine group (4.5 g alanine × 3 times/day). Participants were fed controlled isoenergetic diets with protein intake evenly distributed across three daily meals for diet stabilization. Daily energy requirements were estimated using the Harris-Benedict equation. An activity factor of 1.3 was used during the bedrest period. The findings obtained indicated that while leg lean mass significantly decreased in both groups, leucine supplementation protected knee extensor peak torque more than in the alanine group. Therefore, leucine supplementation appeared to protect muscle health during relatively brief periods of physical inactivity. The parameters of this study allowed for the strict control of diets and nutritional supplementation under energy-matched conditions; therefore, leucine supplementation may help protect muscle function in muscle disuse atrophy.

Holloway et al. examined the safety, tolerability, and atrophy-mitigating effects of a novel amino acid composition (containing essential amino acids and arginine, glutamine, and N-acetylcysteine) during single-limb immobilization [67]. Twenty young men were randomly assigned to receive either the amino acid mixture or an energy-matched, non-amino acid-containing placebo three times a day (two hours after breakfast, lunch, and dinner) for consecutive days. Diets were designed to achieve an energy balance, and meal plans included protein derived from dairy sources held constant at 1.0 g/kg/day. The reduction in the cross-sectional area of the quadriceps muscle was significantly lower in the amino acid group than in the placebo group. However, immobilization resulted in similar relative declines in peak torque in both groups. These findings indicated that the daily consumption of an amino acid mixture (three times a day for 28 days) attenuated muscle atrophy, and are bolstered by the use of well-controlled diets and nutritional supplementation with energy-matched conditions.

A number of human studies examined the effects of nutritional interventions on muscle mass and strength during a period of muscle disuse [68, 69]. Due to insufficient dietary control, these studies were not sufficient to clarify the nutritional value of such supplements. Despite these deficits, many studies have reported the efficacy of nutritional supplementation for preventing the loss of muscle mass and strength during a period of muscle disuse *in vivo* [70–72]. Future studies are needed to clarify whether these candidates for nutritional supplementation preserve muscle mass during disuse. These studies must control diet quality and modify the nutritional intervention period (e.g., expand the duration of nutritional administration before muscle disuse) to provide sufficient evidence.

3. Conclusions

In this chapter, we (a) summarized nutritional epidemiology evidence related to sarcopenia from recent systematic reviews; (b) reviewed the role nutrient supplementation plays in attenuating sarcopenia through dietary control; (c) provided evidence for the efficacy of nutrient supplementation for treating disuse muscle atrophy under controlled diet quality conditions.

a. Dietary patterns of adequate quality for older adults (i.e., ensuring a sufficient intake of beneficial foods, such as fruits, vegetables, whole grain products, fish, nuts, and low-fat foods) are useful for preventing sarcopenia. While the Mediterranean diet has been touted as a healthy diet, other diets (healthy Nordic or traditional Asian diets) also help prevent sarcopenia in older adults.

b. Vitamin D and leucine-enriched whey protein supplement may be useful for attenuating sarcopenia in geriatric patients, particularly in those unable to exercise.

c. Further studies are needed to clarify the effects of protein and amino acid supplementation on muscle mass and strength.

Based on the strong evidence linking nutrition to muscle mass and function, nutrition plays a crucial role in both the prevention and management of sarcopenia. Further high quality studies, particularly those using large sample sizes, controlled diet quality, and iso-caloric placebo supplementation, are needed to provide a clear understanding of the dose and duration effects of nutrients on muscle atrophy.

Conflict of interest

The authors declare no conflict of interest.

Author details

Muneshige Shimizu[1*] and Kunihiro Sakuma[2]

1 Department of Fisheries, School of Marine Science and Technology, Tokai University, 3-20-1 Orido, Shimizu-ku, Shizuoka, Japan

2 Institute for Liberal Arts, Environment and Society, Tokyo Institute of Technology, W9-2, 2-12-1 Ookayama, Meguro-ku, Tokyo, Japan

*Address all correspondence to: shimizu.muneshige@tsc.u-tokai.ac.jp

References

[1] Spahillari A, Mukamal K, DeFilippi C, Kizer JR, Gottdiener JS, Djoussé L, Lyles MF, Bartz TM, Murthy VL, Shah RV: The association of lean and fat mass with all-cause mortality in older adults: the cardiovascular health study. Nutr Metab Cardiovasc Dis. 2016, 26, 1039-1047

[2] Volakilis KA, Halle M, Meisinger C: Muscular strength as a strong predictor of mortality: a narrative review. Eur J Intern Med. 2015, 26, 303-310

[3] Egan B, Zierath JR: Exercise metabolism and the molecular regulation of skeletal muscle adaptation. Cell Metab. 2013, 17, 162-164

[4] Shaw SC, Dennison EM, Cooper C: Epidemiology of Sarcopenia: Determinants Throughout the Lifecourse. Calcif Tissue Int. 2017, 101, 229-247

[5] Cruz-Jentoft AJ, Baeyens JP, Bauer JM, Boirie Y, Cederholm T, Landi F, Martin FC, Michel JP, Rolland Y, Schneider SM, Topinková E, Vandewoude M, Zamboni M; European Working Group on Sarcopenia in Older People. Age Ageing, 2010, 39, 412-423

[6] Sayer AA: Sarcopenia the new geriatric giant: Time to translate research findings into clinical practice. Age Ageing. 2014, 43, 736-737

[7] Dodds RM, Syddall HE, Cooper R, Benzeval M, Deary IJ, Dennison EM, Der G, Gale CR, Inskip HM, Jagger C, Kirkwood TB, Lawlor DA, Robinson SM, Starr JM, Steptoe A, Tilling K, Kuh D, Cooper C, Sayer AA: Grip Strength across the Life Course: Normative data from Twelve British Studies. PLoS ONE. 2014, Dec4, 9(12) e113637

[8] Maynard M, Gunnell D, Ness AR, Abraham L, Bates CJ, Blane D: What influences diet in early old age? Prospective and cross-sectional analyses of the Boyd Orr cohort. Eur J Public Health. 2006, 16, 316-324

[9] Elia M, Russell CA, Stratton RJ: Malnutrition in the UK: Policies to address the problem. Proc Nutr Soc. 2010, 69, 470-476

[10] Margetts BM, Thompson RL, Elia M, Jackson AA: Prevalence of risk of undernutrition is associated with poor health status in older people in the UK. Eur J Clin Nutr. 2003, 57, 69-74

[11] Robinson S, Cooper C, Aihie SA: Nutrition and sarcopenia: A review of the evidence and implications for preventive strategies. J Aging Res. 2012, 2012, 510801

[12] Waijers PM, Feskens EJ, Ocké MC: A critical review of predefined diet quality scores. Br J Nutr. 2007, 97, 219-231

[13] Hu FB: Dietary pattern analysis: A new direction in nutritional epidemiology. Curr Opin Lipidol. 2002, 13, 3-9

[14] Schwingshackl L, Bogensberger B, Hoffmann G: Diet quality as assessed by the healthy eating index, alternate healthy eating index, dietary approaches to stop hypertension score, and health outcomes: An updated systematic review and meta-analysis of cohort studies. J Acad Nutr Diet. 2018, 118, 74-100

[15] Schwedhelm C, Boeing H, Hoffmann G, Aleksandrova K, Schwingshackl L: Effect of diet on mortality and cancer recurrence among cancer survivors: A systematic review and meta-analysis of cohort studies. Nutr Rev. 2016, 74, 737-748

[16] McNaughton SA, Bates CJ, Mishra GD: Diet quality is associated

with all-cause mortality in adults aged 65 years and older. J Nutr. 2012, 142, 320-325

[17] McNaughton SA, Dunstan DW, Ball K, Shaw J, Crawford D: Dietary quality is associated with diabetes and cardio-metabolic risk factors. J Nutr. 2009, 139, 734-742

[18] Robinson SM, Reginster JY, Rizzoli R, Shaw SC, Kanis JA, Bautmans I, Bischoff-Ferrari H, Bruyère O, Cesari M, Dawson-Hughes B, Fielding RA, Kaufman JM, Landi F, Malafarina V, Rolland Y, van Loon LJ, Vellas B, Visser M, Cooper C, ESCEO working group: Does nutrition play a role in the prevention and management of sarcopenia? Clin Nutr. 2018, 37, 1121-1132

[19] Willcox DC, Scapagnini G, Willcox BJ: Healthy aging diets other than the Mediterranean: A focus on the Okinawan diet. Mech Ageing Dev. 2014, 136-137, 148-162

[20] Craig JV, Bunn DK, Hayhoe RP, Appleyard WO, Lenaghan EA, Welch AA: Relationship between the Mediterranean dietary pattern and musculoskeletal health in children, adolescents, and adults: Systematic review and evidence map. Nutr. Rev. 2017, 75, 830-857

[21] Silva R, Pizato N, DaMata F, Figueiredo A, Ito M, Pereira MG: Mediterranean diet and musculo-skeletal-functional outcomes in community-dwelling older people: A systematic review and meta-analysis. J Nutr Health Aging, 2018, 22, 655-663

[22] United Nations: Department of economic and social affairs, population division. world population ageing 2017. http://www.un.org/en/development/desa/ population/publications/pdf/ageing/WPA2017_Highlights.pdf

[23] Steves CJ, Spector TD, Jackson SH: Ageing, genes, environment and epigenetics: What twin studies tell us now, and in the future. Age Ageing 2012, 41, 581-586

[24] Daskalopoulou C, Stubbs B, Kralj C, Koukounari A, Prince M, Prina AM: Physical activity and healthy ageing: A systematic review and meta-analysis of longitudinal cohort studies. Ageing Res Rev. 2017, 38, 6-17

[25] McPhee JS, French DP, Jackson D, Nazroo J, Pendleton N, Degens H: Physical activity in older age: Perspectives for healthy ageing and frailty. Biogerontology 2016, 17, 567-580

[26] Fontana L, Partridge L: Promoting health and longevity through diet: From model organisms to humans. Cell 2015, 161, 106-118

[27] Kiefte-de Jong JC, Mathers JC, Franco OH: Nutrition and healthy ageing: The key ingredients. Proc Nutr Soc. 2014, 73, 249-259

[28] Witard OC, McGlory C, Hamilton DL, Phillips SM: Growing older with health and vitality: A nexus of physical activity, exercise and nutrition. Biogerontology 2016, 17, 529-546

[29] Sofi F, Macchi C, Abbate R, Gensini GF, Casini A: Mediterranean diet and health status: An updated meta-analysis and a proposal for a literature-based adherence score. Pub Health Nutr. 2014, 17, 2769-2782

[30] Deutz NE, Bauer JM, Barazzoni R, Biolo G, Boirie Y, Bosy-Westphal A, Cederholm T, Cruz-Jentoft A, Krznariç Z, Nair KS, Singer P, Teta D, Tipton K, Calder PC: Protein intake and exercise for optimal muscle function with aging: Recommendations from the ESPEN Expert Group. Clin. Nutr. 2014, 33, 929-936

[31] Deer RR, Volpi E: Protein intake and muscle function in older adults. Curr Opin Clin Nutr Metab Care. 2015, 18, 248-253

[32] Beasley JM, Shikany JM, Thomson CA: The role of dietary protein intake in the prevention of sarcopenia of aging. Nutr Clin Pract. 2013, 28, 684-690

[33] Muir SW, Montero-Odasso M: Effect of vitamin D supplementation on muscle strength, gait and balance in older adults: A systematic review and meta-analysis. J Am Geriatr Soc. 2011, 59, 2291-2300

[34] Reedy J, Krebs-Smith SM, Miller PE, Liese AD, Kahle LL, Park Y, Subar AF: Higher diet quality is associated with decreased risk of all-cause, cardiovascular disease, and cancer mortality among older adults. J Nutr. 2014, 144, 881-889

[35] Guasch-Ferre M, Salas-Salvado J, Ros E, Estruch R, Corella D, Fito M, Martinez-Gonzalez MA: The PREMIED trial, Mediterranean diet and health outcomes: How strong is the evidence? Nutr Metab Cardiovasc Dis. 2017, 27 624-632

[36] Schwingshackl L, Hoffmann G: Diet quality as assessed by the healthy eating index, the alternate healthy eating index, the dietary approaches to stop hypertension score, and health outcomes: A systematic review and meta-analysis of cohort studies. J Acad Nutr Diet. 2015, 115, 780-800

[37] Gorman BS, Primavera LH: The complimentary use of cluster and factor analysis methods. J Exp Educ. 1983, 51, 165-168

[38] Robinson SM, Jameson KA, Batelaan SF, Martin HJ, Syddall HE, Dennison EM, Cooper C, Sayer AA, Hertfordshire Cohort Study Group: Diet and its relationship with grip strength in community-dwelling older men and women: The Hertfordshire cohort study. J Am Geriatr Soc. 2008, 56, 84-90

[39] Martin H, Aihie-Sayer A, Jameson K, Syddall H, Dennison EM, Cooper C, Robinson S: Does diet influence physical performance in community-dwelling older people? Findings from the Hertfordshire Cohort Study. Age Ageing 2011, 40, 181-186

[40] Bollwein J, Diekmann R, Kaiser MJ, Bauer JM, Uter W, Sieber CC, Volkert D: Dietary quality is related to frailty in community-dwelling older adults. J Gerontol Ser A Biol Sci Med Sci. 2013, 68, 483-489

[41] Rahi B, Morais JA, Dionne IJ, Gaudreau P, Payette H, Shatenstein B: The combined effects of diet quality and physical activity on maintenance of muscle strength among diabetic older adults from the NuAge cohort. Exp. Gerontol. 2014, 49, 40-46

[42] Hashemi R, Motlagh AD, Heshmat R, Esmaillzadeh A, Payab M, Yousefinia M, Siassi F, Pasalar P, Baygi F: Diet and its relationship to sarcopenia in community dwelling Iranian elderly: A cross sectional study. Nutrition 2015, 31, 97-104

[43] Granic A, Jagger C, Davies K, Adamson A, Kirkwood T, Hill TR, Siervo M, Mathers JC, Sayer AA: Effect of Dietary Patterns on Muscle Strength and Physical Performance in the Very Old: Findings from the Newcastle 85+ Study. PLoS ONE 2016, 11, e0149699

[44] Perala MM, Von-Bonsdorff M, Mannisto S, Salonen MK, Simonen M, Kanerva N, Pohjolainen P, Kajantie E, Rantanen T, Eriksson JG: A healthy Nordic diet and physical performance in old age: Findings from the longitudinal Helsinki Birth Cohort Study. Br J Nutr. 2016, 115, 878-886

[45] Suthuvoravut U, Takahashi K, Murayama H, Tanaka T, Akishita M, Iijima K: Association between traditional Japanese diet washoku and sarcopenia in community-dwelling older adults: findings from the Kashiwa study. J Nutr Health Aging 2020, 24, 282-289

[46] Fung TT, McCullough ML, Newby PK, Manson JE, Meigs JB, Rifai N, Willett WC, Hu FB: Diet-quality scores and plasma concentrations of markers of inflammation and endothelial dysfunction. Am J Clin Nutr. 2005, 82, 163-173

[47] Trichopoulou A, Costacou T, Bamia C, Trichopoulos D: Adherence to a Mediterranean diet and survival in a Greek population. N Engl J Med. 2003, 348, 2599-2608

[48] Shatenstein B, Nadon S, Godin C, Ferland G: Diet quality of Montreal-area adultsneeds improvement: estimates from a self-administered food frequency question-naire furnishing a dietary indicator score. J Am Diet Assoc. 2005, 105, 1251-1260

[49] Moshfegh AJ, Borrud L, Perloff B, LaComb R: Improved method for the 24-hour dietary recall for use in national surveys. FASEB J. 1999, 13, A603

[50] Granic A, Davies K, Adamson A, Kirkwood T, Hill T, Siervo M, Mathers JC, Jagger C: Dietary patterns and socioeconomic status in the very old: the Newcastle 85+ Study. PLoS One 2015, 10, e0139713

[51] Food Standards Agency: McCance and Widdowson's the composition of foods, sixth summary edition. Cambridge, Royal Society of Chemistry 2002

[52] Ronis MJJ, Pedersen KB, Watt J: Adverse effects of nutraceuticals and dietary supplements. Annu Rev Pharmacol Toxicol. 2018, 58, 583-601

[53] Tieland M, van de Rest O, Dirks ML, van der Zwaluw N, Mensink M, van Loon LJ, de Groot LC: Protein supplementation improves physical performance in frail elderly people: a randomized, double-blind, placebo-controlled trial. J Am Med Dir Assoc. 2012, 13, 720-726

[54] Kim CO, Lee KR: Preventive effect of protein-energy supplementation on the functional decline of frail older adults with low socioeconomic status: A community-based randomized controlled study. J Gerontol A Biol Sci Med Sci. 2013, 68, 309-16

[55] Veronese N, Berton L, Carraro S, Bolzetta F, de Rui M, Perissinotto E, Toffanello ED, Bano G, Pizzato S, Miotto F, Coin A, Manzato E, Sergi G: Effect of oral magunesium supplementation on physical performance in healthy elderly women involved in weekly exercise program: a randomized controlled trial. Am J Clin Nutr. 2014, 100, 974-981

[56] Roma KS, Natasza C, Marta L, Ewa Z, Aleksandra S, Janusz W, Katarzyna WT, The effect of a 12-week omega-3 supplementation on bidy composition, muscle strength and physical performance in elderly individuals with decreased muscle mass. Int J Environ Res Public Health 2015, 12, 10558-10574

[57] Bauer JM, Verlaan S, Bautmans I, Brandt K, Donini LM, Maggio M, McMurdo ME, Mets T, Seal C, Wijers SL, Ceda GP, de Vito G, Donders G, Drey M, Greig C, Holmbäck U, Narici M, McPhee J, Poggiogalle E, Power D, Scafoglieri A, Schultz R, Sieber CC, Cederholm T: Effects of a vitamin D and leucine-enriced whey protein nutritional supplement on measures of sarcopenia in older adults, the PROVIDE study: a randomized, double-blind, placebo-controlled trial. J Am Med Dir Assoc. 2015, 16, 740-747

[58] Porter SKN, Pieper CF, Orenduff MC, McDonald SR, McClure LB, Zhou R, Payne ME, Bales CW: Improved function with enhanced

protein intake per meal: a pilot study of weight reduction in frail, obese older adults. J Gerontol A Biol Sci Med Sci. 2016, 71, 1369-1375

[59] Rhoads TW, Clark JP, Gustafson GE, Miller KN, Conklin MW, DeMuth TM, Berres ME, Eliceiri KW, Vaughan LK, Lary CW, Beasley TM, Colman RJ, Anderson RM: Molecular and functional networks linked to sarcopenia prevention by caloric restriction in rhesus monkeys. Cell Syst. 2020, 26, 156-168

[60] Alirezaei M, Kemball CC, Flynn CA, Wood MR, Whitton JL, Kiosses WB: Short-term fasting induced profound neuronal autophagy. Autophagy, 2010, 6, 702-710

[61] Paddon-Jones D, Sheffield-Moore M, Urban RJ, Sanford AP, Aarsland A, Wolfe RR, Ferrando AA: Essential amino acid and carbohydrate supplementation ameliorates muscle protein loss in humans during 28 days bedrest. J Clin Endocrinol Metab. 2004, 89, 4351-4358

[62] Trappe TA, Burd NA, Louis ES, Lee GA, Trappe SW: Influence of concurrent exercise or nutrition countermeasures on thigh and calf muscle size and function during 60 days of bed rest in women. Acta Physiol, 2007, 191, 147-159

[63] Ferrando AA, Paddon-Jones D, Hays NP, Kortebein P, Ronsen O, Williams RH, McComb A, Symons TB, Wolfe RR, Evans W: EAA supplementation to increase nitrogen intake improves muscle function during bed rest in the elderly. Clin Nutr. 2010, 29, 18-23

[64] Deutz NEP, Pereira SL, Hays NP, Oliver JS, Edens NK, Evans CM, Wolfe RR: Effect of beta-hydroxy-beta-methylbutyrate (HMB) on lean body mass during 10 days of bed rest in older adults. Clin Nutr. 2013, 32, 704-712

[65] Dirks ML, Wall BT, Nilwik R, Weerts DHJM, Verdijk LB, van Loon LJC: Skeletal muscle disuse atrophy is not attenuated by dietary protein supplementation in healthy older men. J Nutr. 2014, 144, 1196-1203

[66] English KL, Mettler JA, Ellison JB, Mamerow MM, Arentson-Lantz E, Pattarini JM, Ploutz-Snyder R, Sheffield-Moore M, Paddon-Jones D: Leucine partially protects muscle mass and function during bed rest in middle-aged adults. Am J Clin Nutr. 2016, 103, 465-473

[67] HollowayTM, McGloryC, McKellarS, Morgan A, Hamill M, Afeyan R, Comb W, Confer S, Zhao P, Hinton M, Kubassova O, Chakravarthy MV, Philips SM: A novel amino acid composition ameliorates short-term muscle disuse atrophy in healthy young men. Front Nutr. 2019, 10, 6, 105

[68] Biolo G, Ciocchi B, Stulle M, Bosutti A, Barazzoni R, Zanetti M, Antonione R, Lebenstedt M, Platen P, Heer M, Guarnieri G: Calorie restriction accelerates the catabolism of lean body mass during 2wk of bed rest. Am J Clin Nutr. 2007, 86, 366-372

[69] Johnston APW, Burke DG, Macneil LG, Candow DG: Effect of creatine supplementation during cast-induced immobilization on the preservation of muscle mass, strength, and endurance. J Strength Cond Res. 2009, 23, 116-120

[70] Abe T, Kohno S, Yama T, Ochi A, Suto T, Hirasaka K, Ohno A, Teshima-Kondo S, Okumura Y, Oarada M, Choi I, Mukai R, Terao J, Nikawa T: Soy glycinin contains a functional inhibitory sequence against muscle-atrophy-associated ubiquitin ligase Cbl-b. Int J Endocrinol. 2013, 907565

[71] Asami Y, Aizawa M, Kinoshita M, Ishikawa J, Sakuma K: Resveratrol

attenuates denervation-induced muscle atrophy due to the blockade of atrogin-1 and p62 accumulation. Int J Med Sci. 2018, 3, 628-637

[72] Tabata S, Aizawa M, Kinoshita M, Ito Y, Kawamura Y, Takebe M, Pan W, Sakuma K: The influence of isoflavone for denervation-induced muscle atrophy. Eur J Nutr. 2019, 58, 291-300

Chapter 7

Effects of Physiotherapy Interventions on the Function of the Locomotor System in Elder Age: View of Theory and Practice

Boglárka Debity and Julianna Cseri

Abstract

The aim of this chapter is to give an overview about the aging processes in the neural and muscuo-skeletal system at cellular and tissue level to highlight the demand for physiotherapy interventions. Searching the relevant literature published in the last decade, it was found that the loss of muscle mass (myofiber atrophy and decrease in the number of myofibers) is associated with decreased regeneration capacity of the skeletal muscle, deterioration of the neural control and bone remodeling as well as the impaired microcirculation leading to insufficient adaptation to the physical exercises. In the management of the aging-related deterioration of the skeletal muscle (sarcopenia), the first tool is the resistance training that improves the muscle mass and power as well as the functional outcomes regarding the mobility and physical performance. The endurance (aerobic) training improves the cardiovascular and respiratory status providing better blood supply to the skeletal muscle and exerts some effects directly to the skeletal muscle and bone (increases the mitochondrial functions, improves the bone remodeling). The combination of aerobic and resistance training seems to be more effective against the sarcopenia and osteopenia. The balance training gives additional benefits, so (together with increased muscle power and performance) improves the quality of life.

Keywords: skeletal muscle, skeleto-neuro-muscular system, aging, physiotherapy practice, physiotherapy and aging

1. Introduction

The homeostasis of the neuromuscular system requires preserved muscle structure and functionality with normal regeneration capacity as well as the intact motor control including peripheral innervation and upper control mechanisms. For the normal locomotion the healthy bone structure and function provide stable basis for muscle function and the proper blood supply is inevitable. All components may be influenced by aging and diseases to some extent causing dysfunction of motor activity.

The skeletal muscle fibers are multinucleated huge cells containing contractile proteins (actin and myosin) organized into sarcomeres. In the fetal life the embryonal myoblasts fuse into long multinucleated structures. It is relevant to our topic that the skeletal muscle fibers are categorized basically into slow type (Type I) and fast type (Type II) twitch fibers based on the kinetics of contraction-relaxation cycle and metabolic properties. Recently, this simple model has become more complex and the diversity of muscle fibers has revealed [1].

The skeletal muscle fibers do not show spontaneous activity without innervation. The somatic motor nerves form neuromuscular junction NMJ) with the endplate of the muscle fibers. The NMJ serves as the site of communication between the two structure. One motor neuron commonly innervates more than one muscle fibers constructing a motor unit in which the muscle fibers work together. The motor neurons and the muscle fibers influence the activity of each other, i.e. the motor neuron activates the myofibers, and the muscle fibers release cytokines that act on the motor neuron. The third component of the communication is the perisynaptic Schwann cell (PSC) population. The PSCs play stabilizer and trophic role in the NMJ. Recently, a new component, kranocyte has discovered that is a fibroblast-like cell covering the NMJ. The kranocytes may play role in the post-injury nerve regeneration [2].

The muscle stem cells (satellite cells) are responsible for the muscle repair after a cell damage caused by micro- or macro-traumatization. The satellite cells are located along the multinucleated muscle fibers between the muscle fiber and the basal lamina. On the adequate stimulation they can proliferate, fuse and form a new muscle fiber or – undergoing an asymmetric cell division – can regenerate the pool of the satellite cells [3]. Our knowledge about the factors regulating the normal function of the stem cells and the pathomechanism of impaired muscle repair in different conditions is ever-increasing and reported in many publications. Recently, Feige et al. [4] has reviewed the factors affecting the self-renewal capacity and repairing function of satellite cells in diseases and aging.

The healthy bone is a fundamental organ in the skeletomuscular system. There is an interesting concept to explore the crosstalk between the muscles and the bones. It means that the skeletal muscles and bones interact with each other and keep the homeostasis in normal stage [5]. The bone is a very dynamic structure with continuous bone resorption and counteracting bone formation. This process is called bone remodeling that plays important role in the bone homeostasis. The resident cells of the bone tissue are osteoblasts, osteocytes, osteoclasts and the bone lining cells originated from the mesenchymal stem cells located in the bone marrow. The osteoblasts are responsible for the bone formation characterized by intensive protein synthesis and release of proteins into the bone matrix. The osteocytes located in the lacunae surrounded with the mineralized bone matrix serve as mechanosensors coordinating the function of osteoblasts and osteoclasts. Osteoclasts are multinucleated cells with bone resorptive ability. Recently, information about their cytokine releasing activity and effects on other bone cells has emerged. Bone lining cells are quiescent osteoblasts covering the bone surfaces. Their role in the bone remodeling is poorly understood, but more and more data about their secretory activity and effects on the other bone cells has been published [6–8].

The microcirculation comprises terminal arteriole, arteriovenous capillary, metarteriole, capillary bed and postcapillary venule. The microcirculation supplies the tissues with oxygen and nutrients, delivers carbon-dioxide and metabolic products and provides optimal milieu for cellular functions. Hendrickse and Degens reviewed the morphology and function of microvasculature including the role of these elements in the plasticity of skeletal muscle microcirculation. The adaptation of microcirculation to functional demand is an essential requirement for proper functioning of the muscle. The parallel change in the myofiber diameter and capillary density has been reported in many articles. The endothelial cells are very important in vascular homeostasis and vascular adaptation. Nitric oxide (NO) promotes the release of the vascular endothelial growth factor (VEGF) that serves as the main angiogenetic molecule [9].

Another review article provides an overview on the systemic and local control of blood flow in the skeletal muscle microvasculature. The metabolic and endothelial regulations must be emphasized in relation to the topic of this chapter. The endothelium-derived relaxing (NO, endothelium-derived relaxing factor – EDRF, prostacyclin) or contracting (endothelin) substances play substantial role in the functional adaptation of microcirculation in normal and pathological states. Differences of microcirculation in oxidative and glycolytic muscles are also reviewed that worth to be considered in training protocols [10].

It is generally accepted that the physiotherapy (including various types of exercises) is a key factor in the management of sarcopenia. Basically, the physical exercises can be categorized into endurance (aerobic) and resistance type exercises. The endurance (aerobic) training works with large muscle groups, being sustained and rhythmic, e.g. swimming, burst walking, dancing, cycling, jogging, long distance running, etc. The most prominent functional outcome of this type of exercises is the improvement of the cardiorespiratory functions. The resistance training includes series of movements performed against static or dynamic resistances (e.g. weight, elastic band) that impacts also the major muscle groups and several joints. Usually it is repeated 2 or 3 times per week with increasing dosage. The primary aim of the resistance training is to improve the muscle power as functional outcome [11].

The aim of this chapter is to offer an overview about the aging processes in different elements of the locomotor system, to summarize the current results related to the physiotherapeutic interventions, and to give an insight into the undergoing processes influenced by exercises.

2. Aging-related alteration of the neural and musculo-skeletal system

In the past decade numerous evidences have been accumulated about the structural and functional changes during the aging process in muscle homeostasis including the loss of muscle mass and/or strength, the impaired repair mechanism and the disturbed adaptation of microvasculature to the metabolic demand. The loss of muscle muss and strength (sarcopenia) as well as the decrease in the bone mass (osteopenia, osteoporosis) together with the alteration of cardiovascular and respiratory system and disturbed metabolism cause the frailty syndrome [5, 12]. The regulation of muscle metabolism, its adaptation to nutrition and short-term or chronic physical exercise in young versus elder age have been overviewed in a recent review [13]. Further reviews also provide complex approach to aging process regarding the elements of muscle homeostasis (muscle fibers, motor unit, regenerative capacity, metabolic background) [14, 15].

To interpret the data, it is worth to distinguish the primary and secondary aging. The primary aging of skeleto-neuro-muscular system is manifested in a progressive deterioration in the structure and disturbed function. The secondary aging refers to the additional structural and functional changes caused by diseases and lifestyle factors. The aim of the therapeutic interventions can be to make slower the aging by limiting the secondary aging process [16].

2.1 Aging of skeletal muscle fibers and the whole motor units

Sarcopenia is the progressive loss of muscle mass and/or strength with consequent decline in functional outcome and activity of daily living (ADL) functions.

Among others, Wilkinson et al. [17] reviewed the characteristic changes in the skeletal muscle in elder age. It was revealed that the decline in the muscle mass derives from the muscle fiber atrophy and the decrease in the number of muscle fibers. The imbalance between the protein anabolism and catabolism was detected with conclusion that the protein turnover is mainly affected by the protein intake and the physical activity. The aged muscles seem to be resistant to the anabolic stimulation (e.g. insulin resistance) that causes loss of muscle proteins, i.e. atrophy. The sedentary lifestyle and the chronic, partial immobilization due to physical inactivity facilitate the loss of muscle mass [13, 17].

The impaired mitochondrial functions, mitochondrial dynamics and mitochondrial autophagy with consequent decrease in oxidative capacity of muscles are also associated with the aging-related sarcopenia, especially in the fast type myofibers [18].

A new approach is the investigation of the aging-related changes in the whole motor unit (motor neuron, NMJ and the innervated muscle fibers) together. We have found two review articles reported in the last decade that are closely related to our topic and give an excellent basis for interpretation of the effects of physical exercise on the neuromuscular functions [19, 20].

The loss of motor neurons, formation of very large motor units during reinnervation together with the decrease in the number and diameter of the muscle fibers (sarcopenia) impact negatively the mechanical performance and the fine motor control of the muscles. In the peripheral nervous system, the loss of motor neurons with high diameter is prominent, to large extent in the lumbar region. The effect of aging is muscle specific, i.e. the muscles in the lower limb are more affected than in the upper limb, the muscles being fast (type II) are more impaired than the muscles containing mainly slow fibers (type I). The upper motor control is also impaired by aging due to decreased excitability of corticospinal pathways [19].

The reorganization of the motor units, the decreased number of motor neurons and the increased number of myofibers innervated by an individual motor neuron seems to be the first step in the aging process. At cellular level, decrease in the rate of axoplasmic transport, the velocity of impulse propagation, and the speed of nerve regeneration were detected together with the fragmentation of the NMJ and impaired signal transduction [20].

The impaired neuromuscular function is manifested in the decreased maximum strength, power, and RFD (rate of force rise: DF/Dt) and in the attenuated functional capacity in daily living [19].

2.2 Aging-related decrease in the regeneration capacity of the skeletal muscle

It is widely accepted in the literature that the number of satellite cells with proliferative ability becomes progressively decreased in elder age resulting in the attenuated hypertrophy during exercise and the muscle regeneration after a muscle injury. The impaired self-renewal capacity has also been described in elder age leading to decreased number of satellite cells being in quiescence and become activated under stimulation. The imbalance between the symmetric and asymmetric cell division (resulting in proliferating cells and satellite cells returning to quiescent state) seems to be the key factor in the aging process of the muscle regeneration [3, 4].

The regeneration capacity can be influenced by the intrinsic and extrinsic factors determining the proliferation and differentiation of the satellite cells and the renewal of the quiescent satellite cell pool [21]. The extrinsic factors have been intensively studied [see ref. 4], but the intrinsic mechanisms occurring inside the muscle cells have been rather unknown. Blau et al. reviewed genetic experiments oriented to discover the intrinsic changes in satellite cells associated with aging [22].

In another review the aging-associated genetic changes are also reported. The stem cells become fragile with increasing chance of damage and death. The number of senescent cells (alive, metabolically active cells without cell division) increases that release pro-inflammatory cytokines with consequent inflammation. Replacing the lost myofibers, fibrosis and accumulation of adipose tissue is also characteristic in aging [23].

The first step in the muscle regeneration is the local inflammation when macrophages (M1 and M2) infiltrate the surroundings and eliminate the cell fragments. In elder age, the balance between the M1 and M2 macrophages is impaired leading to improper satellite cell activation. The extracellular matrix is also affected leading not proper milieu for satellite cells [24].

2.3 Aging and bone

The aging process of the bone is manifested in osteopenia and decreased mineralization of the bone (osteoporosis), in a disease with high prevalence and risk of pathologic fractures. The aging of bone (osteopenia) is frequently associated with sarcopenia therefore the physiotherapy interventions must be focused on treatment of sarcopenia and the osteoporosis parallel.

It has been reported recently that the dysfunction of osteogenic mesenchymal stem cells (MSCs) is the one sign of the aging process. The differentiation of MSCs is shifted towards adipogenesis instead of osteogenesis. The details of pathomechanism at cellular and molecular level has been reviewed by Infante and Rodríguez in 2018 [25].

The aging alters the number and function of osteoblasts (bone-forming cells) and causes impaired mineralization. In the background, the impaired organization of the cytoskeletal structure of the osteoblasts is supposed. The accumulation of the free oxygen radicals may be the reason of consequent series of altered processes [26].

In elder age, the adaptation of bone macro- and microstructure to the mechanical load is substantially impaired, mainly due to the inadequate control of osteoblasts and osteoclasts activity by the osteocytes as mechanosensors. Osteocytes are responsible for the balance between the activity of osteoblasts and osteoclasts (bone formation and bone resorption). In the elder age, the osteoclast activity exceeds the osteoblast activity mainly due to the impaired coordinator function of osteocytes. The current literature is heterogenous related to the changes in the density and morphology of osteocytes, the shape of lacunae and canaliculi network. Differences may derive from species and sex differences as well as from different techniques used for measuring and analyzing the data. The type of bone (trabecular or compact) also may modify the changes and reactions of cellular elements [27].

2.4 Aging-related changes in the microcirculation

Evidences for the microcirculatory theory of aging has recently been reviewed. Decreased capillary density with reduced blood flow and insufficient tissue perfusion has been reported by several authors. Although, the experimental data are somehow conflicting according to the basal flow and post-exercise hyperemia in human leg; some evidences exist showing that the blood flow and reactivity of the vessels to exercise decline in elder age [9, 28]. It is suggested that the decrease in the capillary density precedes the sarcopenia [9]. Other data are not in agreement with this statement since neither capillarization nor arrangement of microvasculature seems to be affected by aging, but there are evidences for impaired endothelial functions including decreased NO and prostacyclin production and insufficient spread of vasodilation alone the microvasculature [10].

It is widely accepted that the function of microvasculature is altered by aging itself and due to the accompanying diseases being frequently present in elder people. However, the possibility for *in vivo* investigation of microvasculature is limited by technical difficulties. A new promising tool is the contrast-enhanced ultrasound (CEUS) method that provides a relatively non-invasive imaging technique for clinical and research application [29]. By using this technique, impaired micro- vascular reaction to isometric exercise and attenuated, delayed post-exercise hyperemia were found in middle-aged subjects in comparison to young people without significant differences in vascular morphology and total leg perfusion [30].

Regarding the blood supply, the capillary:fiber (C:F) ratio is a determining parameter. The C:F ratio is lower in the patients with sarcopenia than in the patients at similar age without sarcopenia. The C:F ratio is mainly affected by aging in the skeletal muscle type II (fast) while is not changed in the muscles type I (slow). On the other hand, the increase in the fiber size (hypertrophy) is not associated to the increased capillarization [9].

It is also interesting that the capillary endothelium and the satellite cells act on each other, i.e. the vascular endothelium-derived growth factor (VEGF) stimulates the proliferation of the satellite cells and the angiogenesis is facilitated by the satellite cells. It is reported that the VEGF production is decreased in advanced age leading to loss of capillaries. Furthermore, the distance between the capillaries and satellite cells increases resulting in impaired regeneration of muscle fibers [9].

3. Physiotherapy on functional outcomes

It is widely accepted in the literature that the level of daily physical activity and the structured exercises contribute to the preservation of skeletal muscle structure and function and attenuates the aging-related decline acting directly on the neuromuscular or indirectly on the other system of organs, especially on the cardiorespiratory system [31].

The endurance (aerobic) exercises provide good basis for intervention against the decrease in muscle loss, while resistance exercises directly increase the muscle mass and performance. The combined training programs including resistance and aerobic exercises, completed with balance training provide the effective interventions in prevention of fall and improving the every-day functionality [9].

3.1 Effects of resistance training

The aging causes severe limitation in the every-day physical activity (walking, climbing stairs, rising from a chair etc.), predominantly in the lower extremities. To increase the physical performance, the improvement of the muscle power (the product of muscle force and contraction velocity) is the most important requirement. The widely used traditional resistance training (consisting heavy weights moved at a slow/moderate velocity) increases the power and functional performance but improves the contraction velocity to less extent than the power training (where the concentric movements are performed at high velocities). The power training with rating of perceived exertion is recommended to reach the best functional outcome [31].

The complex effects of strength (resistance) training has also been reviewed including improvement of muscle strength, reduction of sarcopenia and bone loss, as well as decrease in the risk of fall and injury by using different training parameters. Higher intensity of strength training results in more benefits even in old people. Significant improvement of functional and clinical outcomes was found also in patients suffering with different diseases [32]. The relationships between the sarcopenia and physical activity were analyzed in a systematic review and meta-analysis where the resistance training was emphasized as a potent intervention against sarcopenia [33].

In a recent review, the controlled resistance training has been designated as the most powerful and fundamental tool for improvement of muscle strength, power and functional outcomes as gait speed, Timed Up and Go test (TUG), sit-to-stand test, Short Physical Performance Battery (SPPB) scores leading to a decrease in the risk of falls even in the frail persons [9].

Decline in the muscle power begins in the 4th–5th decades, so it is very important to start the progressive resistance training in middle age focusing on the muscles in lower extremity (gluteal muscles, quadriceps, and hamstrings) to prevent the further deterioration and progressive limitations in mobility. The leg press and knee extensor training resulted in similar improvement in the muscle power and functional outcomes. The exercise intensity seems not to be a significant moderator of the efficacy of resistance training improving the muscle force. It is suggested that the higher training intensity results in increase in the absolute force while the training at lower intensity increases the contraction velocity. The training volume (product of sets and repetition) has been in negative correlation with muscle power (the less volume resulted in higher power). The effect of variation in intensity and volume requires further meta-analysis [34].

Another systemic review and meta-analysis revealed that the most effective resistance training regarding the muscle strength was done with 2–3 session/week with 2–3 sets/exercise and 7–9 repletion at 70–79% of the 1RM for 50–53 weeks [35].

The multiple benefits of resistance training were reviewed including the facilitation of the physical functions and increasing the bone mineralization [36].

A follow-up study carried out in 6th and 18 months after a 12-week resistance training with 149 participants explored that the maintenance of benefits gained during a supervised resistance training was sustained only for a short period. 66% of participants self-reported doing the recommended level of physical activity (≥30 min/d) including walking, swimming, gymnastics and gardening, but only less than half of the participants continued the resistance exercises. The muscle strength of quadriceps decreased in comparison to the value at the end of the supervised training but remained higher than before the training program. In general, neither the leisure time physical activity nor the uncontrolled exercise training could completely prevent the decline in the muscle strength, only could limit the negative tendency. In contrast, the result of timed up and go test improved by exercise training was unchanged during the follow-up [37].

Recent review focused on the effect of physical activity in the prefrail or frail persons. Definition of frailty syndrome can be seen in a review article [12]. Although the intervention protocols were heterogenous, the most authors applied resistance training aiming to increase the muscle strength in frailty syndrome. It was generally reported that the physical activity reduced the frailty, improved the physical performance and caused a slight increase in the muscle strength [38].

Comparison of machine-based RT (M-SRT) on stable surface and RT on unstable surface (URT) either in machine-based (M-URT) or free-weight URT (F-URT) form resulted in similarly significant improvement in the muscle strength and power of lower extremities and balance in the groups of old participants (65 to 80 years). The lower extremity muscle strength was increased to highest extent in machine based URT, but the degree of muscle power improvement was independent on the form of exercises. The gait analysis revealed also important impact on parameters independently of the form of training. It has clinical relevance that the maximal training load of the squat-movement was significantly lower in F-URT in comparison to two other types of exercises [39].

3.2 Effects of endurance training

The numerous benefits of endurance (aerobic) training in old age are evidenced in several publications. Regarding the locomotor system, the increased aerobic capacity must be emphasized, but there are evidences for increased muscle strength on the effect of a long-term aerobic training [18].

The impact of endurance training on sarcopenia has been revealed less than of resistance training because the improvement of muscle mass and strength by resistance training is in the focus of investigators [13].

The primary aim of the endurance (aerobic) training is the improvement of cardiovascular functions. Beside the impact on the cardiovascular health the aerobic physical activity influences the metabolism, increases the glucose tolerance, positively acts on body composition, and is an important factor in maintenance of the bone density [40].

3.3 Effects of combined training

There are a lot of publications regarding the effects of combined (multimodal) exercises on general fitness and especially the improvement of sarcopenia in old age. We summarize here the most relevant data gained from supervised, controlled exercise training programs consisting of aerobic (AT) and resistance training (RT) or RT and balance training. The functional outcomes are highlighted beside the feasibility and safety of the programs in old population without sever comorbidities.

Combined AT (2 times/week) and RT (2 times/week) were applied in a 6-week high-volume, moderate-intensity exercise program where the measurement of the functional outcomes (TUG test and the SPPB) was completed with the exploration of feasibility and safety of the training program for old untrained persons. The results showed unchanged TUG but significantly improved SPPB scores. The positive feedback about the subjective experiences during the follow-up in the semi-structured interviews and adherence to enter a longer program indicate that this exercise protocol is promising for the future and worth to consider these findings in planning the exercise interventions [40].

The functional outcomes (gained from the TUG test, the functional reach test, 30-second chair stand test and the 6-minute walk test) were analyzed comparing to the control on the effect of a 32-week aerobic training alone (3 times per week) or combined with resistance training (1 session of RT + 2 session of AT) in a randomized controlled trial carried out in a group of old (˃65ys) men (n = 22 in each group). It was found that the AT alone caused significant decrease in the time measured by TUG test and increase in the value of functional reach test and distance in the 6-minute walk test at the 24th weeks of the program and later. The combined training evoked greater improvement in parameters mentioned above with earlier manifestation (the walking distance became significantly higher as in the control group already at the 8th week). It was suggested by the authors that the improved functional outcomes might decrease the risk of fall [41].

The frequency (2 or 3 times per week) of combined (resistance and aerobic) training did not influence the functional outcomes in old men [42].

It was found in a randomized clinical trial (LIFE study) that the risk of fall in elder age cannot be attenuated by using resistance and balance training together with long-term structured physical activity (walking, strength and balance training) in the very old age (70–89 yeas) in sedentary people with functional limitations, but can reduce the rate of fall with consequent fracture and hospitalization, especially in men. The training program lasted for 24–42 months, partly in a supervised form (2 sessions/week with 63% attendance) and partly in the form of home-based activity (3–4 sessions/week) [43].

The effect of combined, high level balance and moderate intensity resistance training in long-term residential age care was also reported focused on the prevention of fall. Significant decrease in the rate of falls and increase in physical performance were found after a 25-week intervention period with progressive dosage followed by a maintenance program with low dosage up to 12 months [44].

4. Theoretical interpretation of practical experiences

It is interesting to see the theoretical findings regarding the effects of physical exercises on the structure and function at cellular and tissue level. These data may prove evidences for practical experiences and can help to design the training protocols.

4.1 Effect of physical exercise on the muscle itself and the whole motor unit

It is evidenced that the aerobic exercise improves the mitochondrial functions, the synthesis of insulin receptor and the myosin heavy chain protein even in the advanced age [13–15]. Impairment of the mitochondrial structure and function seems to be the consequence of decreased physical activity in older persons rather than the aging itself [14]. Not only the structured physical exercises, but the regular physical activity in the daily life promotes the mitochondrial protein synthesis [45].

It is generally accepted, that the resistance training increases the muscle mass and strength, although, some data show controversary results or the variability of the degree of improvement. The contractile properties of a single muscle fiber seem to be increased by both resistance and endurance training [14]. It is worth to mention that the skeletal muscle reacts to the resistance training in elder age less than younger age, due to the impaired protein synthesis [19].

The studies revealed differences in the remodeling of the muscle fibers on the effect of concentric (CON RET) vs. eccentric resistance training (ECC RET) at the 80% of one-repetition maximum for 4 weeks. Both type of training evoked hypertrophy and increased protein content of the muscles, while the CON RET increased the pennation angle and the ECC RET increased the myofiber length. It is suggested that the new sarcomeres are coupled in parallel to the old ones after a CON RET training but in series by using an ECC RET [46].

It is interesting, that not only the high-load but the low-load resistance exercise can stimulate the mitochondrial biogenesis and function besides the positive effects on the contractile machinery [47].

The electrical stimulation increases the size of the fast type muscle fibers parallel to the decrease in the diameter of the slow type myofibers, similarly to the resistance training in a 70y old population [48].

Although, the aging-related loss of motor neurons seems to be inevitable but physical exercise, especially the strength training can evoke adaptive changes in the motor units that compensate the decrease in the number of motor neurons. The reinnervation of deinnervated muscle fibers by the collateral axons can be promoted, but other data contradict to these findings [19].

Similar findings have recently been reported showing that the muscle cross-sectional area (CSA) in vastus lateralis has decreased by aging independently of different trainings. The number of motor units has been larger in young power training group compared to young controls but in elder age neither the power nor the endurance training have impacted this parameter The size of motor units has increased by age without significant effect of power or endurance training. In conclusion, the benefit of regular training may be the improvement in motor unit remodeling [49].

The power training (concentric contractions at high velocity) evokes earlier activation and higher firing rate in the motor unit [31]. Overview of the spinal motor neuron plasticity, i.e. its adaptation to different exercises has recently been published. In human investigations, indirect approach has been used to get information about the motor neuron behavior analyzing the response of the motor unit by using surface or intramuscular electromyography. The heterogenous training protocols make difficult to explore and interpret the association between the exercise features and the motor neuron response, so this field is open for further investigations [50].

4.2 Effect of physical exercise on the regeneration capacity of the skeletal muscles

Both the short- and long-term resistance training downregulate the M1 type and upregulate the M2 type macrophage expression. This shift facilitates the phagocytosis and satellite cell activation after an injury of muscle fibers improving the regeneration capacity of the skeletal muscle. The electric stimulation increases the number of Pax7 and neural cell adhesion molecule (NCAM) positive satellite cells (myogenic cells committed to differentiation) [48].

It is worth to consider that the mode of contraction used in a resistance training affects the muscle cell damage and regeneration at different way and to different extent. The eccentric muscle contractions (ECC) resulted in higher degree of damage than the concentric ones. The inflammatory cytokine concentration was increased due to the eccentric, but not the concentric exercises. The number of satellite cells increased in ECC group but remained unchanged after the concentric exercises [51]. The eccentric contractions stimulate the production of collage type I, III and IV so restoring the extracellular matrix around the satellite cells. The fibrosis and adipogenesis seems to be attenuated [52].

It has been reported that the number of type I specific Pax7+ satellite cells has increased 96 h after resistance training alone or combined with endurance training but the number of type I specific MyoD+ (activated) cells have increased only after the resistance training. The number of type II specific satellite cells (Pax7+ and MyoD+) have not changed in any type of exercise in vastus lateralis of the middle-aged, overweight/obes, sedentary patients [53].

4.3 Effect of physical exercise on the bone

The loss of muscle mass and strength (sarcopenia) is frequently associated with the impaired structure (osteoporosis) and function of the bone (osteopenia).

Due to the technical difficulties in human (lack of non-invasive technique to measure the mechanical strain in the bone) there are no direct data about the effect of various types of physical exercises on bone cells. The indirect data derive from the measuring the markers for bone formation and bone resorption. The weight-bearing exercises (jumping, aerobics and running) and low impact exercises (as walking) are recommended in several authors and authorities for the prevention of bone loss. However, the effectiveness and feasibility of different trainings seems to be age dependent. In old age the concomitant diseases (joint and cardiovascular problems) make limitation in the choice of training type [54].

A recent publication has revealed a close correlation between the effect of a 3-month combined resistance and weight-bearing training on the bone remodeling and the muscle power in post-menopausal women. The number of circulating osteogenic cells has increased parallel to the bone-formation marker with significant correlation to the one-repetition maxim in the lower and upper extremities [55].

The osteoblast activity showed marked (but not significant) increase on the effect of a 10-week progressive aerobic training in women suffering from postmenopausal osteoporosis [56].

4.4 Effect of physical exercise on the skeletal muscle microcirculation

In advanced age, the reactivity of microcirculation to various factors, especially the endothelium derived relaxing and contracting factors as well as the sympatholytic mechanisms during exercise are impaired. The vasodilation is reduced, and the vasoconstriction is higher than in younger people leading to lower blood flow and decreased tolerance to aerobic exercises [57].

According to the microcirculation theory of aging [28], the impairment of the microvasculature structure and reactivity in old age plays important role in deterioration of the neuromuscular homeostasis and can be an important target for physiotherapy interventions.

Endurance exercises stimulate the angiogenesis and oxidative metabolism in the muscle fibers, so it is recommended to precede the muscle mass increasing resistance exercises [9]. The better capillarization as a result of the long-term aerobic exercises or chronic electric stimulation usually precedes the increased activity of oxidative enzymes. Heavy resistance training does not stimulate the capillarization [10].

5. Recommendations to practitioners

The types of physical activity being feasible even in hospitalized and physically frail patient have been reviewed recently. Resistance exercises alone or in combination with other types of physical activity even done in bed at low to moderate intensity evoke positive changes in the physical performance. High speed, dynamic resistance exercise with concentric contractions are preferable in this situation. Resistance exercises performed by using elastic bands result in significant improvement in muscle power and functional outcome even in a short-term training program. Aerobic exercises with progressive duration (e.g. cycle-ergometer, treadmill or so simple exercises as steps-up, stationary cycling, walking) are strongly recommended [58].

The recently published position statement from the National Strength and Conditioning Association gives an excellent guideline for practitioners engaged in care of old people. Regarding the resistance training protocols directed to old people 2–3 sets of exercises acting on the large muscle groups and many joints with frequency of 2–3 sessions/week at 70–85% of 1RM and inclusion of power exercise with concentric movement at high velocity but moderate intensity (40–60% of 1RM) are recommended. There is a need to adapt the training program to neuromuscular disorders, limitation in movement, the comorbidities and frailty. The completion of resistance training with endurance and balance training is recommended to reach as benefits as possible [59].

The international practice guideline for sarcopenia elaborated by the participants in International Conference on Sarcopenia and Frailty Research strongly recommends the resistance training program for old persons based on evidences. It is noted that the individually tailored training program can be better than the group training but there is some cost limitation for this type of training program. The authors note that increase in physical activity in the leisure time is also advantageous [60].

The combination of aerobic and resistance training is also preferred by other authors to reach the possible maximal functional outcomes [5, 18, 53]. The best effects can be supposed if the aerobic training precedes the resistance training supporting the metabolic adaptation of neuromuscular system [9].

6. Conclusions

The main characteristics of the aging of skeleto-neuro-muscular system at cellular and tissue level is overviewed in a holistic approach with the aim of giving a theoretical basis for physiotherapeutic interventions. The muscle fiber atrophy and numeric decline in the muscle fibers are associated with the fundamental alteration of the motor neurons and NMJ accompanied by the remodeling of motor units. The regeneration capacity of the muscle fibers is attenuated due to the intrinsic aging of the satellite cells and the self-renewal ability of stem cell pool. The aging of neuromuscular system (sarcopenia) is frequently associated with the aging processes in the bone (osteopenia). The blood supply to the skeletal muscle is also affected by the aging of microvasculature leading to decreased vasodilation and increased vasoconstriction responses.

The implementation and functional outputs of resistance and endurance training is overview in the mirror of current literature. It is generally accepted that the resistance training is the most important interventions in the elder age with taking into consideration the aging-dependent limitations. Feasibility and safety relations are also cited. The endurance training alone improves the cardiovascular fitness with lower (but not zero) direct impact on muscle power and performance. The combined training (AT+RT) completed with the elements of balance training seems to be the more effective in old people. The data about the effects of the physical exercises at cellular and tissue level offer good background to interpretation of the practical experiences.

Based on the current literature, we recommend the combined exercise trading, fundamentally based on resistance training but completed with the endurance and balance training elements.

Conflict of interest

The authors declare no conflict of interest.

Author details

Boglárka Debity[1] and Julianna Cseri[2]*

1 University of Debrecen, UDAC Basketball Academy, Debrecen, Hungary

2 University of Debrecen, Department of Physiotherapy, Debrecen, Hungary

*Address all correspondence to: cseri.julianna@gmail.com

References

[1] Schiaffino S, Reggiani C: Fiber types in mammalian skeletal muscles. Physiol Rev. 2011;91(4):1447-531. DOI: 10.1152/physrev.00031.2010.

[2] Lepore E, Casola I, Dobrowolny G, Musarò A: Neuromuscular junction as an entity of nerve-muscle communication. Cells. 2019;8(8): 906. DOI: 10.3390/cells8080906.

[3] Dumont NA, Bentzinger CF, Sincennes MC, Rudnicki MA: Satellite Cells and Skeletal Muscle Regeneration. Compr Physiol. 2015;5(3):1027-59. DOI: 10.1002/cphy.c140068.

[4] Feige P, Brun CE, Ritso M, Rudnicki MA: Orienting muscle stem cells for regeneration in homeostasis, aging, and disease. Cell Stem Cell. 2018;23(5):653-664. DOI: 10.1016/j.stem.2018.10.006.

[5] Greco EA, PietschmannP, Migliaccio S: Osteoporosis and Sarcopenia Increase Frailty Syndrome in the Elderly. Front Endocrinol (Lausanne). 2019;10: 255. DOI:10.3389/fendo.2019.00255.

[6] Sims NA, Vrahnas C: Regulation of cortical and trabecular bone mass by communication between osteoblasts, osteocytes and osteoclasts. Arch Biochem Biophys. 2014;561:22-8. DOI: 10.1016/j.abb.2014.05.015.

[7] Florencio-Silva R, Rodrigues da Silva Sasso G, Sasso-Cerri E, Simões MJ, Cerri PS: Biology of bone tissue: structure, function, and factors that influence bone cells. Biomed Res Int. 2015;2015:421746. DOI: 10.1155/2015/421746.

[8] Katsimbri P: The biology of normal bone remodelling. Eur J Cancer Care (Engl). 2017;26(6):e12740. DOI: 10.1111/ecc.12740.

[9] Hendrickse, P, Degens H: The role of the microcirculation in muscle function and plasticity. J Muscle Res Cell Motil. 2019;40:127-140. https://doi.org/10.1007/s10974-019-09520-2.

[10] Hudlicka O: Microcirculation in skeletal muscle. Muscles Ligaments Tendons J. 2011; 1(1): 3-11.

[11] Lopez P, Pinto RS, Radaelli R, Rech A, Grazioli R, Izquierdo M, · Cadore LS: Benefits of resistance training in physically frail elderly: a systematic review. Aging Clin Exp Res. 2018;30(8):889-899. DOI: 10.1007/s40520-017-0863-z.

[12] Xue QL: The frailty syndrome: definition and natural history. Clin Geriatr Med. 2011;27(1):1-15. DOI: 10.1016/j.cger.2010.08.009.

[13] Brook MS, Wilkinson DJ, Phillips BE, Perez-Schindler J, Philp A, Smith K, Atherton PJ: Skeletal muscle homeostasis and plasticity in youth and ageing: impact of nutrition and exercise. Acta Physiol (Oxf). 2016;216(1):15-41. DOI: 10.1111/apha.12532.

[14] Distefano G, Goodpaster BH: Effects of Exercise and Aging on Skeletal Muscle. Cold Spring Harb Perspect Med. 2018;8(3): a029785. DOI: 10.1101/cshperspect.a029785.

[15] McCornick R, Vasilaki A: Age-related changes in skeletal muscle: changes to life-style as a therapy. Biogerontology 2018;19:519-536. DOI: 10.1007/s10522-018-9775-3.

[16] Cartee GD, Hepple RT, Bamman MM, Zierath JR: Exercise Promotes Healthy Aging of Skeletal Muscle. Cell Metab. 2016;23(6):1034-1047. DOI: 10.1016/j.cmet.2016.05.007.

[17] Wilkinson DJ, Piasecki M, Atherton PJ: The age-related loss of skeletal muscle mass and function: Measurement and physiology of muscle

fibre atrophy and muscle fibre loss in humans. Ageing Res Rev. 2018;47:123-132. DOI: 10.1016/j.arr.2018.07.005.

[18] Yoo S-Z, No M-H, Heo JW, Park D-H, Kang J-H, Kim SH, Kwak H-B: Role of exercise in age-related sarcopenia. J Exerc. Rehabil. 2018;14(4):551-558. DOI: 10.12965/jer.1836268.134.

[19] Aagaard P, Suetta C, Caserotti P, Magnusson SP, Kjaer M: Role of the nervous system in sarcopenia and muscle atrophy with aging: strength training as a counter measure. Scand J Med Sci Sports 2010;20:49-64.

[20] Larsson L, Degens H, Li M, Salviati L, Lee YI, Thompson W, Kirkland JL, Sandri M: Sarcopenia: Aging-Related Loss of Muscle Mass and Function. Physiol Rev. 2019;99(1):427-511. DOI: 10.1152/physrev.00061.2017.

[21] Sousa-Victor P, Muñoz-Cánoves P: Regenerative decline of stem cells in sarcopenia. Mol Aspects Med. 2016;50:109-17. DOI: 10.1016/j.mam.2016.02.002.

[22] Blau HM, Cosgrove BD, Ho ATV: The central role of muscle stem cells in regenerative failure with aging. Nat Med. 2015;21(8): 854-862. DOI: 10.1038/nm.3918.

[23] Parker MH: The altered fate of aging satellite cells is determined by signaling and epigenetic changes. Front Genet. 2015;6: 59.

[24] Perandini LA, Chimin P, da Silva Lutkemeyer D, Olsen N, Câmara S: Chronic inflammation in skeletal muscle impairs satellite cells function during regeneration: can physical exercise restore the satellite cell niche? FEBS J. 2018;285(11):1973-1984. DOI: 10.1111/febs.14417.

[25] Infante A, Rodríguez CI: Osteogenesis and aging: lessons from mesenchymal stem cells. Stem Cell Res Ther. 2018;9(1):244. doi: 10.1186/s13287-018-0995-x.

[26] Lai P, Song Q, Yang C, Li Z, Liu S, Liu B, Li M, Deng H, Cai D, Jin D, Liu A, Bai X: Loss of Rictor with aging in osteoblasts promotes age-related bone loss. Cell Death and Disease. 2016);7: e2408. DOI:10.1038/cddis.2016.249.

[27] Hemmatian H, Bakker AD, Klein-Nulend J, van Lenthe GH: Aging, Osteocytes, and Mechanotransduction. Curr Osteoporos Rep. 2017;15:401-411. DOI 10.1007/s11914-017-0402-z

[28] Jin K: A Microcirculatory Theory of Aging. Aging Dis. 2019;10(3): 676-683. DOI: 10.14336/AD.2019.0315.

[29] Dunford EC, Au JS, Devries MC, Phillips SM, MacDonald MJ: Cardiovascular aging and the microcirculation of skeletal muscle: using contrast-enhanced ultrasound. Am J Physiol Heart Circ Physiol 2018;315: H1194–H1199. DOI: 10.1152/ajpheart.00737.2017.

[30] Hildebrandt W, Schwarzbach H, Pardun A, Hannemann L, Bogs B, König AM, Mahnken AH, Hildebrandt O, Koehler U, Kinscherf R: Age-related differences in skeletal muscle microvascular response to exercise as detected by contrast-enhanced ultrasound (CEUS). PLoSONE 2017;12(3):e0172771. DOI:10.1371/journal. pone.017277.

[31] Tiggemann CL, Dias CP, Radaelli R, Massa JC, Bortoluzzi R, Wolf Schoenell MC, Noll M, Alberton CL, Martins Kruel LF: Effect of traditional resistance and power training using rated perceived exertion for enhancement of muscle strength, power, and functional performance. Age (Dordr). 2016;38(2):42. DOI: 10.1007/s11357-016-9904-3.

[32] Mayer F, Scharhag-Rosenberger F, Carlsohn A, Cassel M, Müller S, Scharhag J: The Intensity and Effects of

Strength Training in the Elderly. Dtsch Arztebl Int. 2011;108(21):359-364. DOI: 10.3238/arztebl.2011.0359.

[33] Steffl M, Bohannon RW, Sontakova L, Tufano JJ, Shiells K, Holmerova I: Relationship between sarcopenia and physical activity in older people: a systematic review and meta-analysis. Clin Interv Aging. 2017;12:835-845. DOI: 10.2147/CIA.S132940.

[34] Straight CR, Lindheimer JB, Brady AO, Dishman RK, Evans EM: Effects of Resistance Training on Lower-Extremity Muscle Power in Middle-Aged and Older Adults: A Systematic Review and Meta-Analysis of Randomized Controlled Trials. Sports Med. 2016;46(3):353-64. DOI: 10.1007/s40279-015-0418-4.

[35] Borde R, Hortobágyi T, Granacher U: Dose-Response Relationships of Resistance Training in Healthy Old Adults: A Systematic Review and Meta-Analysis. Sports Med. 2015;45(12):1693-720. DOI: 10.1007/s40279-015-0385-9.

[36] Westcott WL: Resistance training is medicine: effects of strength training on health. Curr Sports Med Rep. 2012;11(4):209-16. DOI: 10.1249/JSR.0b013e31825dabb8.

[37] Geirsdottir OG, Arnarson A, Ramel A, Briem K, Jonsson PV, Thorsdottir I: Muscular strength and physical function in elderly adults 6-18 months after a 12-week resistance exercise program. Scand J Public Health 2014;43(1):76-82. DOI:10.1177/1403494814560842.

[38] Haider S, Grabovac I, Dorner TE: Effects of physical activity interventions in frail and prefrail community-dwelling people. Wien Klin Wochenschr. 2019;131(11): 244-254. DOI: 10.1007/s00508-019-1484-7.

[39] Eckardt N: Lower-extremity resistance training on unstable surfaces improves proxies of muscle strength, power and balance in healthy older adults: a randomised control trial. BMC Geriatr. 2016;16(1):191. DOI: 10.1186/s12877-016-0366-3.

[40] Falck RS, Davis JC, Milosevic E, Liu-Ambrose T: How much will older adults exercise? A feasibility study of aerobic training combined with resistance training. Pilot Feasibility Stud. 2017;3:2. DOI: 10.1186/s40814-016-0116-5.

[41] Sousa N, Mendes R, Silva A, Oliveira J: Combined exercise is more effective than aerobic exercise in the improvement of fall risk factors: a randomized controlled trial in community-dwelling older men. Clin Rehabil. 2017; 31(4):478-486. DOI: 10.1177/0269215516655857.

[42] Ferrari R, Fuchs SC, Kruel LF, Cadore EL, Alberton CL, Pinto RS, Radaelli R, Schoenell M, Izquierdo M, Tanaka H, Umpierre D: Effects of Different Concurrent Resistance and Aerobic Training Frequencies on Muscle Power and Muscle Quality in Trained Elderly Men: A Randomized Clinical Trial. Aging Dis. 2016;7(6):697-704. DOI:10.14336/AD.2016.0504.

[43] Gill TM, Pahor M , Guralnik JM , McDermott MM, King AC, Buford TW, Strotmeyer ES, Nelson ME, Sink KM, Demons JL, Kashaf SS, Walkup MP, Miller ME, LIFE Study Investigators: Effect of structured physical activity on prevention of serious fall injuries in adults aged 70-89: randomized clinical trial (LIFE Study). BMJ. 2016;352:i245. DOI: 10.1136/bmj.i245.

[44] Hewitt J, Goodall S, Clemson L, Henwood T, Refshauge K: Progressive Resistance and Balance Training for Falls Prevention in Long-Term Residential Aged Care: A Cluster Randomized Trial of the Sunbeam Program. J Am Med Dir Assoc. 2018;19(4):361-369. DOI: 10.1016/j.jamda.2017.12.014.

[45] Ubaida-Mohien C, Gonzalez-Freire M, Lyashkov A, Moaddel R, Chia CW, Simonsick EM, Sen R, Ferrucci L: Physical Activity Associated Proteomics of Skeletal Muscle: Being Physically Active in Daily Life May Protect Skeletal Muscle from Aging. Front Physiol. 2019;10:312. DOI: 10.3389/fphys.2019.00312.

[46] Franchi MV, Reeves ND, Narici MV: Skeletal Muscle Remodeling in Response to Eccentric vs. Concentric Loading: Morphological, Molecular, and Metabolic Adaptations. Front Physiol. 2017;8:447. DOI:10.3389/fphys.2017.00447.

[47] Groennebaek T, Vissing K: Impact of resistance training on skeletal muscle mitochondrial biogenesis, content, and function. Front. Physiol. 2017;8:713. DOI: 10.3389/fphys.2017.00713.

[48] Zampieri S, Mosole S, Löfler S, Fruhmann H, Burggraf S, Cvečka J, Hamar D, Sedliak M, Tirptakova V, Šarabon N, Mayr W, Kern H: Physical Exercise in Aging: Nine Weeks of Leg Press or Electrical Stimulation Training in 70 Years Old Sedentary Elderly People. Eur J Transl Myol. 2015;25(4):237-42. DOI: 10.4081/ejtm.2015.5374.

[49] Piasecki M, Ireland A, Piasecki J, Degens H, Stashuk DW, Swiecicka A, Rutter MK, Jones DA, McPhee JS: Long-Term Endurance and Power Training May Facilitate Motor Unit Size Expansion to Compensate for Declining Motor Unit Numbers in Older Age. Front Physiol. 2019;10:449. DOI: 10.3389/fphys.2019.00449.

[50] Button DC, Kalma JM: Understanding exercise-dependent plasticity of moto neurons using intracellular and intramuscular approaches. Appl Physiol Nutr Metab. 2019;44(11):1125-1133. DOI: 10.1139/apnm-2018-0862.

[51] Hyldahl RD, Olson T, Welling T, Groscost L, Parcell AC: Satellite cell activity is differentially affected by contraction mode in human muscle following a work-matched bout of exercise. Front Physiol. 2014;5:485. DOI: 10.3389/fphys.2014.00485.

[52] Perandini LA, Chimin P, Lutkemeyer D, Câmara N: Chronic inflammation in skeletal muscle impairs satellite cells function during regeneration: can physical exercise restore the satellite cell niche? FEBS J. 2018;285(11):1973-1984. DOI: 10.1111/febs.14417.

[53] Pugh JK, Faulkner SH, Turner MC, Nimmo MA: Satellite cell response to concurrent resistance exercise and high-intensity interval training in sedentary, overweight/obese, middle-aged individuals. Eur J Appl Physiol. 2018;118(2): 225-238. DOI: 10.1007/s00421-017-3721-y.

[54] Troy KL, Mancuso ME, Butler TA, Johnson JE: Exercise Early and Often: Effects of Physical Activity and Exercise on Women's Bone Health. Int J Environ Res Public Health. 2018;15(5):878. DOI: 10.3390/ijerph15050878.

[55] Pasqualini L, Ministrini S, Lombardini R, Bagaglia F, Paltriccia V, Pippi R, Collebrusco L, Reginato E, Sbroma Tomaro E, Marini E, D'Abbondanza M, Scarponi AM, De Feo P, Pirro M: Effects of a 3-month weight-bearing and resistance exercise training on circulating osteogenic cells and bone formation markers in postmenopausal women with low bone mass. Osteoporos Int. 2019;30(4):797-806. DOI: 10.1007/s00198-019-04908-9.

[56] Wen HJ, Huang TH, Li TL, Chong PN, Ang BS: Effects of short-term step aerobics exercise on bone metabolism and functional fitness in postmenopausal women with low bone mass. Osteoporos Int. 2017;28(2):539-547. DOI: 10.1007/s00198-016-3759-4.

[57] Hearon Jr CM, Dinenno FA: Regulation of skeletal muscle blood flow during exercise in ageing humans. J Physiol. 2016;594(8): 2261-2273. DOI: 10.1113/JP270593.

[58] Valenzuela PL, Morales JS, Pareja-Galeano H, Izquierdo, Emanuele E, de la Villa P, Lucia A: Physical strategies to prevent disuse-inducted functional decline int he elderly. Ageing Res Rev 2018; 47:80-88. DOI: 10.1016/j.arr.2018.07.003.

[59] Fragala MS, Cadore EL, Dorgo S, Izquierdo M, Kraemer WJ, Peterson MD, Ryan ED: Resistance Training for Older Adults: Position Statement from the National Strength and Conditioning Association. J Strength Cond Res. 2019;33(8):2019-2052. DOI: 10.1519/JSC.0000000000003230.

[60] Dent E, Morley JE, Cruz-Jentoft AJ, et al: International Clinical Practice Guidelines for Sarcopenia (ICFSR): Screening, Diagnosis and Management. J Nutr Health Aging. 2018;22(10):1148-1161. doi:10.1007/s12603-018-1139-9

Chapter 8

Total Antioxidant from Herbal Medicine as a Possible Tool for the Multifunctional Prevention of Muscular Atrophy

Viani Anggi

Abstract

Muscular atrophy is one of disease by the loss of skeletal muscle mass. So, by the loss in muscle often causes rapid muscle atrophy and the occurs during injury and illness its causes immobilization in spinal muscle mass. Usually, the impact factor of the nervous system in musculoskeletal is caused by aging, immobility, malnutrition, medication and even the range of injuries disease impact by the nervous system. To meet the needs needed by the loss of skeletal, we need high total antioxidant from herbal medicine as multifunctional potentially prevention of muscular atrophy condition. Antioxidants are agents that can slow down or prevent oxidation process and protect cells system from the damage of cell by the loss skeletal in muscle mass. One of herbal medicine is *Abelmoschus manihot* L. Medik From Palu of central Sulawesi as a possible multifunctional prevention of Muscular Atrophy, where the total antioxidant value is 3,45 mg/mL.

Keywords: total antioxidant, herbal medicine, multifunctional prevention, muscular atrophy

1. Introduction

Muscular atrophy is one of disease by the loss of skeletal in muscle mass. The muscular atrophy recessive autosomal in neuromuscular with characterized of alpha motor neuron in the spinal cord [1]. The neuromuscular disorders are one factor genetic of infant mortality [2]. The spinal muscular atrophy deletion or mutation the Survival motor neuron 1 (SMN 1 gene), reduction of levels functional survival motor neuron 1 (SMN 1 gene) and also resulting selective death of spinal motor neurons system in a pathway, it's depends by the age of onset, symptoms and maximum function achieved [3]. By the age at the onset it causes at birth: Neuromuscular disease, congenital myotonic dystrophy and spinal muscular atrophy, other causes are systematic septicemia-induced disease, lung damage, intracranial pathologies, infection of the central nervous system, disorders of the peripheral nerves, disease of the neuromuscular junction, Prader-Willi syndrome and drug intoxication during pregnancy or delivery system and after 6 months of age were the neuromuscular disease: spinal muscular atrophy types II and III, polyneuropathies, childhood myasthenia gravis, muscular dystrophies and metabolic myopathy and besides that in other causes were congenital heart disease, malnutrition, rickets, metabolic diseases, nephropathies and lung diseases [4, 5]. The clinical prognosis of

IntechOpen

spinal muscular atrophy is variable and depends on types of spinal muscular atrophy continuous spectrum with the age of death by infancy to normal life expectancy condition system on cell pathway system [6]. The Muscular atrophy its described with characterized generalized muscle and atrophy in the proximal limb muscle and phenotype by four grades of severity, where the spinal Muscular Atrophy I, spinal Muscular Atrophy II, spinal Muscular Atrophy III and spinal Muscular Atrophy IV, it's all depended by onset and motor spinal function [7, 8]. The muscular atrophy disease by the control mutation in the homozygous of survival motor neuron α (SMN 1) gene. The skeletal of muscular atrophy it's adverse consequences and the mechanism such as wasting or decrease of injury time. Lack of use in the spinal muscular atrophy and event disease category of spinal muscular atrophy. The spinal muscular atrophy it's usually considered by chronic diseases such as poliomyelitis, Diabetes mellitus, cancer, renal failure or pulmonary obstruction [1].

To activation of spinal muscular atrophy, we need the process to activation of the distinct pathway (ATP) in proteolysis pathway. The condition of spinal muscular atrophy it's depends on the level of muscle protein nutrition system. To reduce the fiber muscle we need synthesis protein to innervate proximal hindlimb muscles and medical motor neurons axial muscles [9]. Mitochondrial is important in skeletal muscle to activation of function and subpopulation involved in cellular functions. Mitochondria play in role key on muscle fibers to the regulation of myonuclear apoptosis and serving uptake the calcium [10]. Mitochondria also continuously produce superoxide radicals and dismutated into hydrogen peroxide (H_2O_2), where H_2O_2 is a relatively and diffuse freely with cytosol, it's very important as signaling to the molecule on cell, to affecting multiple control of the cell cycle, uptake to cellular stress response, activation energy metabolism and also to the expression of numerous redox-sensitive genes in spinal muscular atrophy disease [9].

2. Prevalence, incidence and carrier frequency of muscular atrophy

According to the worldwide about a study into the prevalence and incidence of spinal muscular atrophy, where approximately 1–2 per 100.000 people and incidence around 1 in 10.000 live births have been estimated with the spinal muscular atrophy type I accounting for around 60% of all cases and estimation of the incidence of all types of spinal muscular atrophy of around 10 in 100.000 (1 in 10.000) live birth is cited [11]. Every incidence is a factor from a number of new cases of the disease in a particular time period. The evaluation of the incidence of all type SMA combined it's around 8 per 100.000 live births. The incidence of spinal muscular atrophy type I is around 4–6 in 100.000 and for the type II and III it's a high incidence combined 10,6 per 100.000 and for the gender, it's a nearly even split male and female [12]. The indicated difference of spinal muscular atrophy types is the between ethnicities and differences in health system clinically diagnosed. The prevalence in Indonesia of neuromuscular in RSCM hospital from January – December 2017 is 2,6% of all patients who come to the neurology outpatient ward. The five most who have neuromuscular disorders are neuropathy peripheral, Duchenne muscular dystrophy, spinal muscular atrophy, Guillain barre syndrome and chronic inflammatory demyelinating polyneuropathy [13].

3. Genetics of spinal muscular atrophy

Spinal muscular atrophy is a defect in survival motor neuron 1 (SMN 1) and it's gene localized to 5q11.2-q13.3). SMN gene (SMN 1 and SMN 2) on chromosome

5q13 and the homozygous deletion of the SMN 1 gene result in Spinal muscular atrophy. Besides that, the SMN 2 gene it produces mostly a shortened, unstable the survival motor neuron mRNA and also to alternative splicing, a small amount of full – length on functional SMN mRNA. The SMN 2 gene is a good prognostic of the spinal muscular atrophy in clinical severity. The clinical severity management of spinal muscular atrophy disease is supportive to increase the survival motor neuron expression levels in motor neurons cells system. So, the management of spinal muscular atrophy depends on increase SMN expression levels in motor neurons [3].

The survival motor neuron 1 gene it should be sequenced mutations if both full SMN 1 present of diagnosis on spinal muscular atrophy is highly, but the SMN 1 gene should be sequenced if the striking typical phenotype, where if sequencing indicates and intact SMN 1 gene of phenotype suggestive of spinal muscular atrophy neurogenic. The survival motor neuron 2 gene should be routinely assessed and it's important to factor system influencing the severity of the spinal muscular atrophy phenotype [1].

4. Molecular oxidative stress factor of muscular atrophy

Factor oxidative stress of muscle atrophy it's important to maintenance and quality to the rehabilitation of disease. The skeletal of muscle atrophy need continuously produce oxidants like as a reactive oxygen species (ROS) and reactive nitrogen species (RNS) to an imbalance of skeletal muscle mechanism process. The soluble atrophy it's produced different oxidative stress state species such as O_2^-, H_2O_2 and OH^-. Where, it also needs antioxidant species state such as catalase, glutathione peroxidase (GPx) and superoxide dismutase (SOD) and the last to imbalance denominated of oxidative stress, it's can produce oxidative damage in lipids, Deoxyribonucleic acid (DNA) and protein to impairing functional protein factor of cellular system [14].

Generation of ROS could uptake of oxygen, activation of NADPH oxidase and to production of the superoxide anion radical, see the reaction:

$$2O_{2+}\ NADPH \xrightarrow{\text{oxidase}} 2O_2^- + NADP^+ + H^+ \quad (1)$$

Where O_2^- is converted to H_2O_2 (Eq. (2) by SOD

$$2O_{2+}\ 2H^+ \xrightarrow{SOD} H_2O_2 + O_2 \quad (2)$$

The skeletal of muscle atrophy could inactivity increase of mitochondrial reactive oxygen species (ROS) production on the ways. The mitochondrial could uptake of calcium and increase mitochondrial levels state of fatty acid hydroperoxides and the last depressed protein could transport into the mitochondria system. So, if the mechanism responsible, it's could increase mitochondrial fission [9].

The observation of muscle mass-specific overexpression of Peroxisome proliferator-activated receptor-y-coactivator-1α (PGC-1α) and the master regulator of mitochondria biogenesis could prevent activation of catabolic system and disuse of muscle atrophy system. The Peroxisome proliferator-activated receptor-y-coactivator-1α (PGC-1α) is mediated pathway and focuses on the role PGC-1α in the skeletal spinal muscular atrophy system by immobilization system. The Peroxisome proliferator-activated receptor-y-coactivator-1α (PGC-1α) is the master transcription stimulates of mitochondrial biogenesis pathway system with up the regulating system of the nuclear respiratory factors (NRF-1,2) and mitochondrial transcription factor A (Tfam) system, so it leads to increased mitochondrial DNA replication system and gene transcription system [15]. The Peroxisome proliferator-activated receptor-y-coactivator-1α (PGC-1α) to appears key to the role-play a protective against of muscular atrophy linked skeletal muscle deterioration. The Peroxisome proliferator-activated receptor-y-coactivator-1α (PGC-1α) interacts with the nuclear receptors and activate transcription factors to activated their target gene. The activity to responsive multiple stimuli including calcium ion, Reactive oxygen species (ROS) and ATP demand pathway system on the cell system in the spinal muscular atrophy. The metabolic stress mediated by PGC-1α downregulation plays a major role in muscle atrophy and to adaptation the soleus to mice hindlimb unloading (HU) in the defuse, we need antioxidant treatment (Trolox). Which, the HU caused of reduction in the cross-sectional area, redox status alteration (NRF2, Superoxide dismutase1 and catalase up-regulation) and the autophagy (Beclin1 and P62 mRNA up-regulation) [16]. The attractive of PGC-1α states in muscle mass could restore and promote the muscle metabolic system when normal physical activity impossible. The observation of the muscle fiber – specific event until overexpression of the attractive of PGC-1α states, where a master regulator of the mitochondrial biogenesis, to prevent activation produce of the catabolic system and also disuse muscle atrophy.

5. Antioxidant mechanism and function

The natural antioxidant is one important to underlying to spinal muscular atrophy system. The natural antioxidant could effect to exercise the health-promoting increase muscle defenses [17]. The natural antioxidant which role-plays to activation integrity on the cell and to prevent the free radical configuration tissue damage of muscle atrophy to normal healthy condition system of muscle atrophy pathway [18].

The natural antioxidant increasing antioxidative defenses and develop a synthesis of endogenous enzymes or increased antioxidant utilization, practice to maintain optimal body function to especially of spinal muscular atrophy in the redox condition on cell [19]. The function from natural antioxidant: it reduces the free radical of spinal muscular atrophy, stimulates the growth of normal cells, to protects the cell against the premature and abnormal aging condition of spinal muscular atrophy, helps fight the age-related molecular degeneration of spinal muscular atrophy and the last to supports the body immune system [17]. The natural antioxidant is powerful electron donors and also to the reaction of free radicals to target molecules breaking damaged on skeletal muscular. The lipid phase of chain-breaking antioxidant can scavenge the radicals in membranes and lipoprotein particles to preventing lipid peroxidation of skeletal muscular atrophy. The lipid phase such as tocopherols, ubiquinol, carotenoids and flavonoids and the aqueous phase such as ascorbate, urate, glutathione and other thiols [20, 21].

6. Flavonoids are group of antioxidants

Flavonoids are a group from based on natural substances by a variable phenolic structure, where are found from fruits, vegetables, grains, bark, roots, stems, flowers, tea and wine. Flavonoids are potential to anti-oxidative, anti-inflammatory and anti-mutagenic on spinal muscular atrophy disease [22]. As an anti-inflammatory, we need of agent system, where the COX is an endogenous enzyme with catalyzes function, which the conversion of arachidonic acid into prostaglandins and thromboxanes, where the enzyme exists in two isoforms: COX - 1 is a constitutive enzyme and is responsible for the supply of prostaglandin and Cox – 2 is an inducible enzyme and is expressed an inflammatory stimulus and the stimulus prostaglandin to induction of inflammatory and pain. By using, the flavonoids can activate the molecular docking and knowledge bioinformatics in preventing chronic disease like as spinal muscular atrophy and to application and manufacturing in pharmaceutical medicinal industry [23]. Flavonoids subdivided of subgroup depending on the carbon of the C ring on which the B ring, which the degree of unsaturation and oxidation of the C ring. The firs isoflavone, which in the B ring is linked position 3 of the C ring. Second, the neoflavonoids, which the B ring is linked in position 4. Besides that, the subdivided into several subgroups on the basis which the B ring is linked position 2 on the basis of the structural features of the C ring. Flavonol (e.g. Quercetin, myricetin), flavone (eg. apigenin, luteolin), flavonolols (eg. taxifolin), flavan-3-ols (eg catechin, epigallocatechin), flavovone [24] (eg. hesperitin, naringenin), anthocyanidin (eg. cynidin, delphidin), isoflavone (eg. genistein, daidzein).

7. *Abelmoschus manihot* L. Medik is one of herbal medicine

Abelmoschus manihot L. Medik is have highest total antioxidant (**Table 1**). The leaf plant is a tropical plant from china, which is trapped by the name Huangkui. Ethanobotanical uses and phytochemical analysis of *Abelmoschus manihot* L. Medik, where the preliminary study shows the presence of alkaloid, carbohydrates, tannins, steroid and glycosides [25].

Compound		Name
1	Hyperoxide/ Hyperin	Dihydroxyphenil)-3-{3R,4S,5R,6R)-3,4,5-trihydroxy-6(hydroxymethyl) oxan-2-yl}oxy-4H-chromene-4,5,7-triol
2	Isoquercetin	2-(3,4-dihydroxyphenyl)-5,7-dihydroxy-3{(2S,3R,4S,5S,6R)-3,4,5-trihydroxy 6-(hydroxymethyl)oxan-2-yl} oxychromen-4-one
3	Myricetin	3,5,7-Trihydroxy-2-(3,4,5)-trihydroxyphenyl-4-chromenone
4	Hibifolin	quercetin 3-beta-robinobioside; 3{(6–0-(6-Deoxy-alpha-L-mannopryranosyl)-beta-D-galactopyranosyl}oxy)-2-(3,4-dihydroxy phenyl)5,7-dihydroxy-4H-1-benzopyran-4-one
5	Quercetin	3-O-robinoside: Quercetin 3 –beta-robinobioside; 3-{(6-O-(Deoxy-alpha-L-mannopyranosyl)-beta-D-galactopyranosy} oxy)-2-(3,4-dihydroxyphenyl-4H-1-benzopyran-4-one
6	Coumarin scopoletin	7-hydroxy-6-methoxychromen-2-one

Table 1.
Some compounds isolated from the genus Abelmoschus manihot *L. Medik [26].*

8. Ethanomedicinal, phytochemical and pharmacological of *Abelmoschus manihot*

Ethanomedicinal, phytochemical and pharmacological profile of genus *Abelmoschus manihot* L. Medik where the genus *Abelmoschus manihot* L. Medik has been reported to used for several ethnomedicinal practices and also demonstrated diverse pharmacological activities and posses several phytochemical and nutritional properties as well as having and no adverse effect on living cells, their pods, seeds and leaves are reported to be used in pharmaceutical industries and traditional remedies all over the world [26]. The protective effect on the total flavonoid of *Abelmoschus manihot* L. Medik on transient cereberal ischemia-preperfusion injury is due to activation of the Nrf2-are pathway, where the highest total flavonoids 788,56 mg/g) of all the different part, the protective effects of an extract of the total flavonoids of *Abelmoschus manihot* L. Medik on transient cereberal ischemia–reperfusion injury (TCI-RI) were investigated, these data suggest that to protects against TCI-RI by scavengin free radical and activating NRF2-ARF pathway (Nuclear factor E2-related factor 2 contributes to neuroptotective immune system, antioxidation, antifatigue and anti-inflamatory properties [27]. The bioactive compounds from *Abelmoschus manihot* L. Medik alleviate the progression of multiple myeloma in mouse model and improve bone marrow environment, where the *Abelmoschus manihot* L. Medik derived as a Huangkui capsules (HKC) represent a traditional Chinese medicine that has been widely applied to the clinical therapy of kidney and inflamatory disease by methods expressions of certain proteins were detected via western blotting, transcriptomic RNA-sequencing as well as RT-qPCR, where the result revealed that MM-Prone animals appeared to be protected following HKC treatment as evidence by a prolonged survival rate, which four of the nine flavonoid compounds (Hyperin/hyperoxide, HK-2; cannabiscitrin, HK-3, 3-O-kaempferol-3-O-acetyl-6-O-(p-coumaroyl)-β-D-glucopyranosid, HK-11, 8-(2-pyrolidione-5-yl)-3-O-β-D-glucopyranosid, HK-E3) suppressed osteoclastogenesis in murine raw 264.7 cells.HK-11 directly inhibited MM cells (ARP1 and h929) proliferation and induced G0/G1 cell cycle arrest, which may have involved suppressing β-catenin protein, increasing expression of IL-6 and TNF-α, as well as activating mature TGF-β1 and some other metabolic pathways [28]. *Abelmoschus manihot* L. Medik have supplementation as a Nephropathy system by methods a combined treatment of a high – fat diet and streptozotocin after unilateral nephrectomy and supplementation of *Abelmoschus manihot* L. Medik were tested, the results is preventive effects of the extracts on Nephropathy pathology system and changes on autophagy mitocondrial proteins were investigated to showed significant increase in fasting blood glucose, plasma creatinine, blood urea nitrogen and urinary albumin levels [29]. *Abelmoschus manihot* L. Medik as a Huangkui in Chinese, where as a traditional Chinese medicine, the Huangkui has been used for medication of the patients as a reduce inflammation anti-oxidative stress, improving immune response system, protecting renal tubular epithelial cells, ameliorating podocyte apoptosis, glomerulosclerosis and mesangial proliferation, as well as inhibiting on cellular and molecular mechanism [30]. So, with the natural antioxidant as a reduces the free radical of spinal muscular atrophy and stimulates the growth of normal cells. In Palu city of central Sulawesi Indonesia, where the plant is known as one of the raw based material of vegetables and is usually mixed with pulp.

9. Total antioxidant of *Abelmoschus manihot* (L.) Medik

This plant is believed to have medicinal based properties, because are many compound vitamins, like as: A, B1, B2, B3, C and E, compound the calcium, potassium, copper, zinc and many collagen. This plant also contains secondary metabolites like as: Flavonoids, Saponin and phonolite, where it has used as an antioxidant. The evaluate total antioxidant arrest activity using the DPPH (IC_{50}) of *Abelmoschus manihot* (L.) Medik extracts from Palu of Central Sulawesi, the method is displayed in **Table 2** and **Figure 1**, evaluate the potential activity of the test substances for the cytotoxicity against selected 4 T1 cell lines and Vero cell of *Abelmoschus manihot* (L.) Medik extracts from Palu of Central Sulawesi. The

Name of Test Substance	**Antioxidant Activity DPPH IC_{50} (mg/mL)**
Leaf *Abelmoschus manihot* (L.) Medik extract	3,45

Table 2.
The antioxidant activity DPPH (IC_{50}) of leaf Abelmoschus manihot *(L.) Medik [32].*

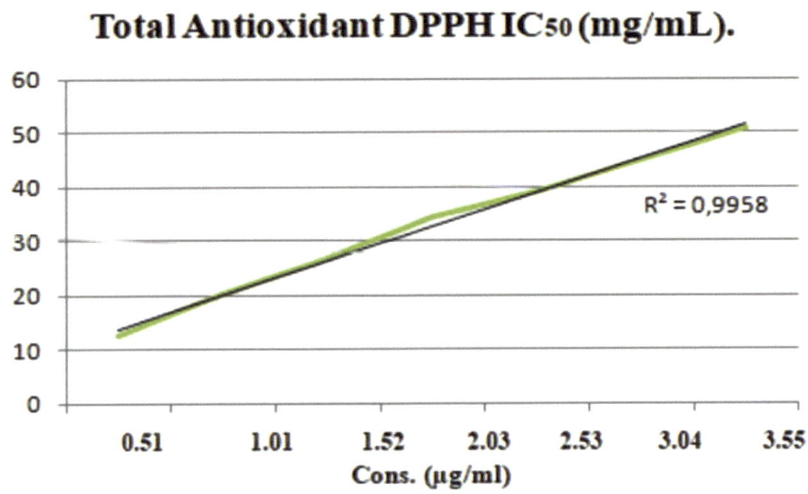

Figure 1.
Graph of total antioxidant of Abelmoschus Manihot.

cytotoxicity potential of various concentration of ethanol, ethyl acetate, N-Heksan extracts with CTC_{50} values of leaf *Abelmoschus manihot* (L.) Medik is displayed in **Tables 3** and **4** and **Figures 2** and **3**. Leaf *Abelmoschus manihot* (L.) Medik from Palu of Central Sulawesi extract plant shows the total antioxidant is 3,45 μg/ml from reports arrest of DPPH (IC_{50}) is displayed in **Table 2** and **Figure 1**. According to the criteria to the level of antioxidant power with DPPH (IC_{50}) method, where the extract of natural ingredients with IC_{50} < 50 μg/ml is potential. The in-vitro cytotoxicity effects of leaf *Abelmoschus manihot* (L.) Medik from Palu of Central Sulawesi, where carried with various concentrations to the breast cancer cell lines 4 T1 and have Potentially Toxicity, where the leaf of *Abelmoschus manihot* (L.) Medik of the medicinal plant was collected from Palu of central Sulawesi and extracted with ethanol solvent with use of Six different concentrations (31.25 μg/ml, 62.5 μg/ml, 125 μg/ml, 250 μg/ml, 500 μg/ml and 1000 μg/ml) of leaf extracts were used to investigate study the in-vitro cytotoxicity concentration potential of the medicinal plant. The cytotoxicity potential of various extracts is N-Heksan extract of *Abelmoschus manihot* (L.) Medik with CTC_{50} values of *Abelmoschus manihot* (L.) Medik is displayed in **Table 3** and **Figure 2**. The results that the cytotoxicity rate has increased when the concentrations of leaf *Abelmoschus manihot* (L.) Medik extracts increases. MTT assay measured the viability cell based on the reduction of yellow tetrazolium MTT to a purple formazan dye by mitochondrial succinate dehydrogenase enzyme. Where the amount of formazan produced reflected the number of metabolically active 4 T1 cells Line (Breast Cancer). The test substances Leaf Extract (ethanol), Leaf Extract (ethyl acetate) and Leaf Extract (N-Heksan) were exhibited a CTC_{50} value of 261.84 ± 0.13 μg/ml, 288.29 ± 0.10 μg/ml and 185.06 ± 0.12 μg/ml. According to the criteria value of the cytotoxicity level of extracts, if an excerpt of natural ingredients with CTC_{50} < 100 μg/ml is very active, the CTC_{50} value of 100–200 μg/ml is quite active and > 200 μg/ml is weak [31]. The

NO	Name of Test Substance	Test Conc. (μg/ml)	% Cytotoxicity	CTC_{50} (μg/ml)
1	Leaf extract (Ethanol)	1000	*83.31 ± 0.003*	261.84 ± 0.13
		500	*73.44 ± 0.014*	
		250	*54.25 ± 0.025*	
		125	*19.93 ± 0.020*	
		62.5	*18.64 ± 0.066*	
		31.25	*2.56 ± 0.049*	
2	Leaf extract (Ethyl Acetate)	1000	66.28 ± 0.016	288.29 ± 0.10
		500	57.02 ± 0.007	
		250	54.45 ± 0.019	
		125	40.81 ± 0.025	
		62.5	28.17 ± 0.011	
		31.25	12.29 ± 0.020	
3	Leaf extract (N-Heksan)	1000	94.45 ± 0.006	185.06 ± 0.12
		500	67.77 ± 0.014	
		250	52.36 ± 0.038	
		125	37.50 ± 0.005	
		62.5	25.33 ± 0.015	
		31.25	16.55 ± 0.017	
4	Doxorubicin	100	68.24 ± 0.007	13.57 ± 0.10
		50	62.50 ± 0.007	
		25	53.51 ± 0.017	
		12.5	47.09 ± 0.109	
		6.25	42.29 ± 0.009	
		3.12	40.00 ± 0.002	

CTC_{50}- Cytotoxicity concentration.

Table 3.
Cytotoxic properties of test substances of leaf Abelmoschus Manihot *(L.) Medik on 4 T1 cell line [32].*

results of N-Heksan leaf extract *Abelmoschus manihot* (L.) Medik has quite potentially to the cytotoxicity. The N-Heksan leaf extract *Abelmoschus manihot* (L.) Medik shows the better percentage of growth inhibition CTC_{50} is 185.06 ± 0.12 μg/ml 4 T1 cell lines. To the Doxorubicin of cytotoxicity CTC_{50} with value 4 T1 cells line is 13,57 ± 0.10 μg/ml, where this value shows is toxic of Doxorubicin to 4 T1 cells Line (Breast Cancer). The cytotoxicity with various concentrations of all leaf extracts does not have potentially the cytotoxicity on Vero (normal) cell, where the cytotoxicity with value $CTC_{50} \geq 200$ μg/ml. The test substances Leaf Extract (ethanol), Leaf Extract (ethyl acetate) and Leaf Extract (N-Heksan), were exhibited a CTC_{50} value of 588.39 ± 0.13 μg/ml, 451.41 ± 0.11 μg/ml and 559.12 ± 0.13 μg/ml. According to the criteria value of the cytotoxicity level of extracts, if an extract of natural ingredients with $CTC_{50} < 100$ μg/ml is very active, the CTC_{50} value of 100–200 μg/ml is quite active and > 200 μg/ml is weak, where is displayed in **Table 4** and **Figure 3**. Results that the cytotoxicity rate has increased when the concentrations of leaf *Abelmoschus manihot* (L.) Medik extracts increases. To the Doxorubicin cytotoxic CTC_{50} value to Vero (normal) cells is 60.85 ± 0.13 μg/ml, this shows is toxic from according to the criteria

No	Name of Test Substance	Test Conc. (μg/ml)	% Cytotoxicity	CTC_{50} (μg/ml)
1	Leaf extract (Ethanol)	1000	57.98 ± 0.051	588.39 ± 0.13
		500	56.43 ± 0.062	
		250	23.33 ± 0.027	
		125	19.74 ± 0.006	
		62.5	9.29 ± 0.006	
		31.25	0.00 ± 0.038	
2	Leaf extract (Etil Acetat)	1000	65.34 ± 0.005	451.41 ± 0.11
		500	54.98 ± 0.003	
		250	38.52 ± 0.006	
		125	25.75 ± 0.002	
		62.5	9.39 ± 0.002	
		31.25	0.77 ± 0.006	
3	Leaf extract (N-Heksan)	1000	68.44 ± 0.005	559.12 ± 0.13
		500	37.07 ± 0.101	
		250	31.55 ± 0.004	
		125	26.42 ± 0.010	
		62.5	12.58 ± 0.056	
		31.25	0.00 ± 0.030	
4	Doxorubicin	100	99.71 ± 0.011	60.85 ± 0.13
		50	94.77 ± 0.005	
		25	84.60 ± 0.065	
		12.5	58.95 ± 0.057	
		6.25	52.95 ± 0.064	
		3.12	37.27 ± 0.008	

CTC_{50}- Cytotoxicity concentration.

Table 4.
Cytotoxic properties of test substances against on Vero cells [32].

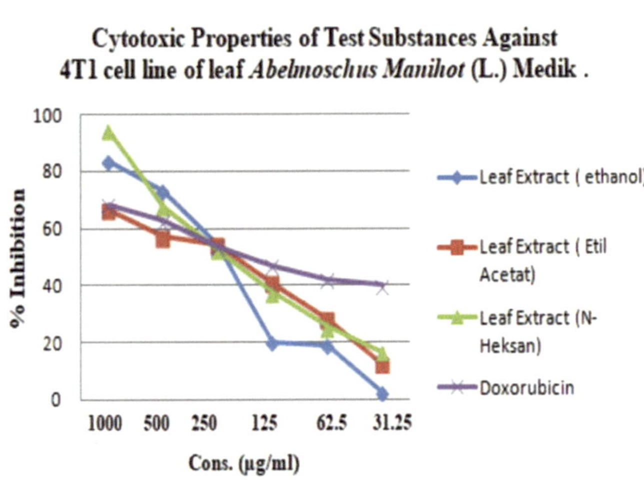

Figure 2.
Graph of cytotoxic effect on 4 T1 cells line of Abelmoschus Manihot *(L.) Medik [32].*

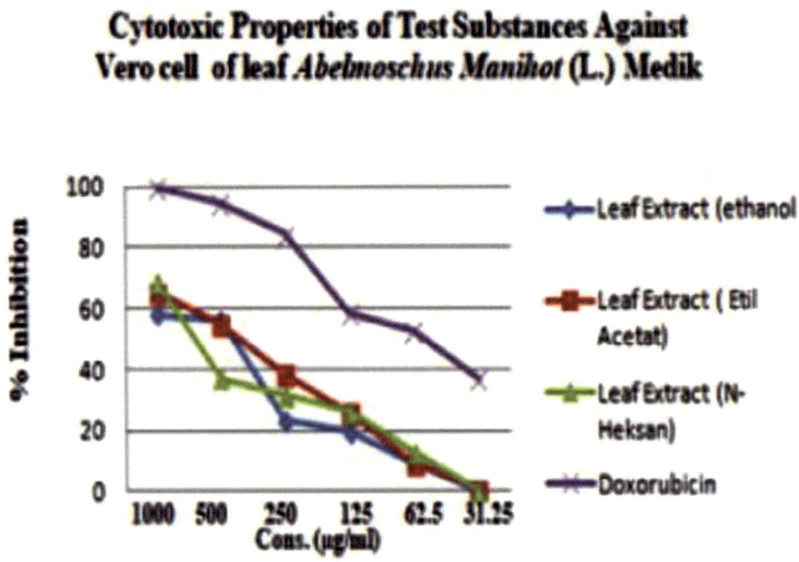

Figure 3.
Graph of the cytotoxic effect of Abelmoschus Manihot *(L.) Medik on Vero cell [32].*

value of cytotoxicity level [32]. The medicinal plant of leaf *Abelmoschus manihot* (L.) Medik from Palu of Central Sulawesi extract, where can be used to prepare the natural antioxidant and to prepare the pharmaceutical-based natural drug with proper standardization methods. Medicinal plants are a source of important therapeutic for alleviating human ailments and the medicinal plants have bioactive compounds, which are used for curing various human disease and also play an essential role key in chronic disease to especially on spinal muscular atrophy cell system pathway [33]. The natural antioxidant as a reduces the free radical of spinal muscular atrophy, stimulates the growth of normal cells, to protects the cell against the premature and abnormal aging condition of spinal muscular atrophy, helps fight the age-related molecular degeneration of spinal muscular atrophy and the last to supports the body immune system [34, 35].

10. Summary

The muscular atrophy recessive autosomal in neuromuscular with characterized of alpha motor neuron in the spinal cord, the neuromuscular disorders is one factor genetic of infant mortality and the spinal muscular atrophy deletion or mutation the Survival motor neuron. Spinal muscular atrophy is a defect in survival motor neuron 1 (SMN 1) and it's gene localized to 5q11.2-q13.3). SMN gene (SMN 1 and SMN 2) on chromosome 5q13 and the homozygous deletion of the SMN 1 gene result in Spinal muscular atrophy. The spinal muscular atrophy disease need of natural antioxidant as a reduces the free radical of the fiber muscle cell, stimulates the growth of normal cells, to protects the cell against the premature and abnormal aging condition of spinal muscle fiber, helps fight the age-related molecular degeneration of spinal muscular cell and the last to supports the body immune system. The medicinal plant of leaf *Abelmoschus Manihot* (L.) Medik from Palu of Central Sulawesi extract, where can be used to prepare the natural antioxidant and to prepare the pharmaceutical-based natural drug with proper standardization methods. Medicinal plants are a source of important therapeutic for alleviating human ailments and medicinal plants have bioactive compounds, which are used for curing various human disease and also play an essential role key in chronic disease to especially on spinal muscular atrophy cell system pathway.

Acknowledgements

Especially Praise the father, praise the Son, praise the spirit three in one God of glory, Majesty praise forever to the King of King my lovely Jesus Christ. But He said to me, "My grace is sufficient for you, for my power is made perfect in weakness (2 Corinthians 12:9).

Conflict of interest

The authors have no conflict of interest.

Author details

Viani Anggi
Department College of Pharmaceutical, Central Sulawesi, 94111, Indonesia

*Address all correspondence to: viani.anggi@gmail.com

References

[1] Mercuri E, Finkel RS, Muntoni F, et al. Diagnosis and management of spinal muscular atrophy: Part 1: Recommendations for diagnosis, rehabilitation, orthopedic and nutritional care. *Neuromuscul Disord*. 2018;28(2):103-115. doi:10.1016/j.nmd.2017.11.005

[2] Teoh HL, Carey K, Sampaio H, Mowat D, Roscioli T, Farrar M. Inherited Paediatric Motor Neuron Disorders: Beyond Spinal Muscular Atrophy. *Neural Plast*. 2017;2017. doi:10.1155/2017/6509493

[3] J. Kolb, Stephen & Kissel JT. Spinal Muscular Atrophy Stephen. *Neurol Clin*. 2015;33(4):831-846. doi:10.1016/j.ncl.2015.07.004.Spinal

[4] Baioni MTC, Ambiel CR. Spinal muscular atrophy: Diagnosis, treatment and future prospects. *J Pediatr (Rio J)*. 2010;86(4):261-270. doi:10.2223/JPED.1988

[5] Yaser salem. Spinal Muscular Atrophy. *Intechopen*. 2012;1(1):13. doi:10.1016/j.colsurfa.2011.12.014

[6] Sumner CJ, Fischbeck KH. Spinal muscular atrophy. *Neurobiol Dis*. 2007;(00168):501-511. doi:10.1016/B978-012088592-3/50046-3

[7] Ewout J.N.Groen KT& THG. Advances in therapy for spinal muscular atrophy: promises and chalenges. *Nat Rev Neurol*. 2018;14(1):214-224.

[8] McKinnell IW, Rudnicki MA. Molecular mechanisms of muscle atrophy. *Cell*. 2004;119(7):907-910. doi:10.1016/j.cell.2004.12.007

[9] Powers SK, Wiggs MP, Duarte JA, Murat Zergeroglu A, Demirel HA. Mitochondrial signaling contributes to disuse muscle atrophy. *Am J Physiol - Endocrinol Metab*. 2012;303(1):31-39. doi:10.1152/ajpendo.00609.2011

[10] Leduc-Gaudet JP, Auger MJ, Jean Pelletier F, Gouspillou G. Towards a better understanding of the role played by mitochondrial dynamics and morphology in skeletal muscle atrophy. *J Physiol*. 2015;593(14):2993-2994. doi:10.1113/JP270736

[11] Verhaart IEC, Robertson A, Wilson IJ, et al. Prevalence, incidence and carrier frequency of 5q-linked spinal muscular atrophy - A literature review. *Orphanet J Rare Dis*. 2017;12(1):1-15. doi:10.1186/s13023-017-0671-8

[12] The John walton. A worldwide study into the prevalence and incidence of spinal muscular atrophy. *Muscular dystrophy Res Cent*. 2015;1(1):12.

[13] Dewi MM, Widodo DP, Amardiyanto R, Sinaga N, Hidayah N. Prevalence, Spectrum Neurofisiologi Neuromuskular case. *Sari Pediatr*. 2019;20(4):214. doi:10.14238/sp20.4.2018.214-20

[14] Abrigo J, Elorza AA, Riedel CA, et al. Role of oxidative stress as key regulator of muscle wasting during cachexia. *Oxid Med Cell Longev*. 2018;2018. doi:10.1155/2018/2063179

[15] Kang C, Ji LL. Role of PGC-1α signaling in skeletal muscle health and disease. *Ann N Y Acad Sci*. 2012;1271(1):110-117. doi:10.1111/j.1749-6632.2012.06738.x

[16] Cannavino J, Brocca L, Sandri M, Bottinelli R, Pellegrino MA. PGC1-α over-expression prevents metabolic alterations and soleus muscle atrophy in hindlimb unloaded mice. *J Physiol*. 2014;592(20):4575-4589. doi:10.1113/jphysiol.2014.275545

[17] Merry TL, Ristow M. Do antioxidant supplements interfere with skeletal muscle adaptation to exercise training? *J Physiol*. 2016;594(18):5135-5147. doi:10.1113/JP270654

[18] Nimse SB, Pal D. Free radicals, natural antioxidants, and their reaction mechanisms. *RSC Adv*. 2015;5(35):27986-28006. doi:10.1039/c4ra13315c

[19] Kurutas EB. The importance of antioxidants which play the role in cellular response against oxidative/nitrosative stress: Current state. *Nutr J*. 2016;15(1):1-22. doi:10.1186/s12937-016-0186-5

[20] Zulaikhah ST. The Role of Antioxidant to Prevent Free Radicals in The Body. *Sains Med*. 2017;8(1):39. doi:10.26532/sainsmed.v8i1.1012

[21] I S Young JVW. Antioxidants in health and disease. *J Clin Pathol*. 2001;54:176-186. doi:10.1201/b18539

[22] Panche AN, Diwan AD, Chandra SR. Flavonoids: An overview. *J Nutr Sci*. 2016;5:1-15. doi:10.1017/jns.2016.41

[23] Wang T yang, Li Q, Bi K shun. Bioactive flavonoids in medicinal plants: Structure, activity and biological fate. *Asian J Pharm Sci*. 2018;13(1):12-23. doi:10.1016/j.ajps.2017.08.004

[24] Li S, Chen G, Zhang C, Wu M, Wu S, Liu Q. Research progress of natural antioxidants in foods for the treatment of diseases. *Food Sci Hum Wellness*. 2014;3(3-4):110-116. doi:10.1016/j.fshw.2014.11.002

[25] Kb A, Ak D, Rn S, Ub A. International Journal of Botany Studies International Journal of Botany Studies Ethanobotanical Uses and Phytochemical analysis of Abelmoschus manihot (L.) Medik. *Int J Bot Stud Int J Bot Stud*. 2018;3(2):149-151. www.botanyjournals.com.

[26] M.M O. Ethnomedicinal, phytochemical and pharmacological profile of genus Abelmoschus. *Phytopharmacology*. 2013;4(3):648-663.

[27] Luo Y, Cui HX, Jia A, Jia SS, Yuan K. The Protective Effect of the Total Flavonoids of *Abelmoschus esculentus* L. Flowers on Transient Cerebral Ischemia-Reperfusion Injury Is due to Activation of the Nrf2-ARE Pathway. *Oxid Med Cell Longev*. 2018;2018:1-11. doi:10.1155/2018/8987173

[28] Hou J, Qian J, Li Z, Gong A, Zhong S, Qiao L, Qian S, Zhang Y, Dou R, Li R, Yang Y GC. Bioactive Compounds from Abelmoschus manihot L. Alleviate the Progression of Multiple Myeloma in Mouse Model and Improve Bone Marrow Microenvironment. *Onco Targets Ther*. 2020;13(1):959-973. https://doi.org/10.2147/OTT.S235944.

[29] Kim H, Dusabimana T, Kim SR, et al. Supplementation of Abelmoschus manihot ameliorates diabetic nephropathy and hepatic steatosis by activating autophagy in mice. *Nutrients*. 2018;10(11):1-16. doi:10.3390/nu10111703

[30] Li N, Tang H, Wu L, et al. Chemical constituents, clinical efficacy and molecular mechanisms of the ethanol extract of Abelmoschus manihot flowers in treatment of kidney diseases. *Phyther Res*. 2020;(March):1-9. doi:10.1002/ptr.6818

[31] Subarnas A, Diantini A, Abdulah R, et al. Antiproliferative activity of primates-consumed plants against MCF-7 human breast cancer cell lines. *J Med Res*. 2012;1(4):38-43.

[32] Anggi V, Adikusuma W. Total antioxidant and in-vitro cytotoxic of

abelmoschus manihot (L.) medik from palu of central sulawesi and doxorubicin on 4t1 cells line and vero cells. *Res J Pharm Technol*. 2019;12(11):5472-5476. doi:10.5958/0974-360X.2019.00949.1

[33] Kasote DM, Katyare SS, Hegde M V., Bae H. Significance of antioxidant potential of plants and its relevance to therapeutic applications. *Int J Biol Sci*. 2015;11(8):982-991. doi:10.7150/ijbs.12096

[34] Dutra MT, Martins WR, Ribeiro ALA, Bottaro M. The Effects of Strength Training Combined with Vitamin C and E Supplementation on Skeletal Muscle Mass and Strength: A Systematic Review and Meta-Analysis. *J Sports Med*. 2020;2020:1-9. doi:10.1155/2020/3505209

[35] Dutra MT, Alex S, Silva AF, Brown LE, Bottaro M. Antioxidant Supplementation Impairs Changes in Body Composition Induced by Strength Training in Young Women. *Int J Exerc Sci*. 2019;12(2):287-296. http://www.ncbi.nlm.nih.gov/pubmed/30899342%0Ahttp://www.pubmedcentral.nih.gov/articlerender.fcgi?artid=PMC6413849.

Chapter 9

Management of Sarcopenic Obesity for Older Adults with Lower-Extremity Osteoarthritis

Tsan-Hon Liou, Chun-De Liao and Shih-Wei Huang

Abstract

Lower-extremity osteoarthritis (OA) is a prevalent musculoskeletal disease in elder population. The main symptom of OA is pain which leads to muscle weakness and physical disability. Recently, muscle weakness, function limitation, and severity of disease in OA are addressed to aging-related muscle attenuations. Therefore, elder individuals with OA are under potential sarcopenia risks. In addition, obesity, which exerts negative impacts on disease outcomes, has become a burden in OA population. Under multifactor risks of OA, it is important to identify effectiveness of multidisciplinary management for such elder population to prevent sarcopenic obesity and maintain physical function. Previous studies have indicated that diet intervention (DI) using protein supplement, dietary protein, or weight loss enhances exercise efficacy in terms of additional muscle mass and strength gains to exercise training (ET) for elder individuals with high sarcopenia and frailty risks. However, it remains unclear whether DI in combination with ET augments any benefit for older adults with lower-extremity OA. This chapter aimed to review the effects of DI plus ET on muscle mass, strength, and physical function outcomes in older individuals with lower-extremity OA.

Keywords: sarcopenia, osteoarthritis, protein supplement, exercise training, muscle mass, function outcome

1. Introduction

Elderly population aged 65 and over is a substantially growing population which is estimated to exceed 16% of global population worldwide in the year of 2050 [1]. Elongation of life expectancy is accompanied with an increase of chronic diseases leading to restricted physical function and disabilities in daily life [2, 3], among which musculoskeletal disorder is a significant public health issue with 7.5–35.2% of the elder people having mild to moderate musculoskeletal conditions [3, 4] and has become the second cause of global burden worldwide compared with other causes of morbidity-mortality [5].

Among the age-related musculoskeletal disorders, osteoarthritis (OA) is one of the most prevalent musculoskeletal diseases from the sixth to the ninth decade of lifespan, especially the OA in lower extremities is closely associated with limitations of functional activities and participation [6]. In addition, sarcopenia, obesity, or in combination of both called sarcopenic obesity have great impacts on physical function in older adults [7, 8]. The impacts of sarcopenia on musculoskeletal system are accounted to the risks of physical limitation in elder individuals, especially those with hip or knee OA [9, 10]. The age-related muscle dysfunction can be addressed to impairments in musculoskeletal system as well as neuromuscular system [11, 12]. With respective to the underlying mechanisms of sarcopenia in older population, muscle atrophy (i.e., decline in muscle size) plays a key role in muscle attenuation [11], especially the type II myofiber [13]. The loss of muscle mass occurs progressively from middle-age by a rate of 0.47% per year in men and 0.37% per year in women [14]; in people aged 75 years, muscle mass is decreased at a rapid rate of 0.64–0.70% per year in women and 0.80–0.98% per year in men and in severe diseases can lead to a loss of approximate 50% by the 8–9th decade of life [15]. Loss of skeletal muscle mass is commonly accompanied with deficits in muscle function such as muscle weakness, which is relevant to clinical presentation of sarcopenia as well as OA. Reid et al. indicated that leg lean mass is strongly associated with muscle strength ($r = 0.78$, $p < 0.01$) [16]. Liu et al. further indicated that low handgrip strength is strongly associated with decreased skeletal muscle mass in elder individuals [17]. Because of that loss of muscle strength may lead to physical difficulty and disability, low muscle mass has been identified as a crucial factor of functional limitation of physical mobility such as walk capability and chair rise [8, 17, 18].

Recently, the disease progression of knee and hip OA has been attributed to age-related decline in muscle mass (i.e., sarcopenia). Toda et al. reported that older women with knee OA experienced significantly lower leg lean mass relative to body weight (%) by a mean ± standard deviation of 19.2 ± 2.7%, compared with the healthy control (21.0 ± 2.9%; $P < 0.0001$) [19]; Lee et al. observed similar results which indicated that older adults with knee OA had a mean appendicular skeletal muscle mass of 15.6 kg which is significant lower than that of healthy control (17.3 kg, $P < 0.001$) [20]. Additionally, Jeon et al. reported that lower skeletal muscle mass independently associated with knee radiographic OA [odds ratio (OR) 1.34; 95% confidence interval (CI) 1.04, 1.75] [21]. Therefore, older people with knee OA are considered at high risk of sarcopenia [22]. Grimaldi et al. observed muscle mass decreased in patients with hip OA in terms of 2.6–14.4% muscle atrophy of gluteal muscle group in the affected side compared to those in the uninvolved side, whereas such asymmetry in muscle volume ranged from 0.4 to 3.7% in control peers [23]; in addition, the muscle volume asymmetry is positively associated with disease progression of hip OA, indicating that patients with moderate to severe OA may experience greater muscle mass loss than mild-severity or asymptomatic patients [24]. Therefore, the OA population faces not only age-related muscle attenuation (i.e., sarcopenia) but also the disease-induced muscle loss.

The sarcopenia, obesity, and OA are becoming major threats to aging society and have been recognized as important health issues [8, 25–27]. The relationships among sarcopenia, obesity (i.e., sarcopenic obesity), and OA have been discussed. Kemmler et al. conducted an observational study to investigate the prevalence of sarcopenia in community-dwelled women who aged 70 years and older; the results indicated that elder women with lower-extremity OA exhibited a significantly higher rate of sarcopenia (9.1%) than nonarthritic peers (3.5%) [28]. Jin et al. reported that elder men and women with sarcopenic obesity showed significantly higher risks of exhibiting knee OA (OR = 1.92–2.43) compared with the healthy control groups [29]. Misra et al. conducted a longitudinal study of the risk of radiographic OA in relation to sarcopenic obesity; the result showed that elder people with sarcopenic obesity (RR = 1.91) had increased risks of exhibiting knee OA within a 5-year interval of follow up [30]. Therefore, preventive efforts for the obese elder individuals may need to focus not only on reducing sarcopenia but also on improving sarcopenic obesity to reduce the growing incidence and prevalence of knee OA.

2. Treatments and management for sarcopenia in elderly

Sarcopenic obesity originates from a multifactorial consequence of aging and its related physical inactivity [31], which especially exerts negative impacts to obese elderly populations [32]. Several approaches for management of sarcopenic obesity have been recommended including pharmacological interventions, exercise interventions, and nutrition interventions to counteract muscle loss and physical declines in obese older adults [33]. According to the recommendations from the European Society for Clinical Nutrition and Metabolism Expert Group [34], there are urgent needs for elder people with a risk of sarcopenic obesity to incorporate nutrition intervention and muscle strengthening exercise to prevent the functional decline.

2.1 Protein supplement plus exercise training for sarcopenic obesity

Obesity has become epidemic burden in elderly population [25]. Sarcopenic obesity, a recently identified phenotype of obese elderly population, is developed based on an underling additive effect of sarcopenia and obesity and is referred by the coexistence of diminished muscle mass and increased fat mass. Sarcopenia has been characterized by age-related muscle degeneration [35], and obesity with an increased body fat exerts negative impacts on the skeletal muscle turnover and its homeostasis [31]. Such deteriorations of muscle mass loss originated from aging process result in muscle dysfunction which may further lead to physical deficits in frail elderly [36]. Furthermore, older adults who are identified as overweight or obesity have been observed suffering high risks of physical disability [37, 38]. Accordingly, sarcopenic obesity had been identified to be associated with more physical limit than either pure sarcopenia or obesity and was served as a risk to disability and frail life style [8, 39]. Therefore, the preservation of muscle mass and strength are vital for obese older adults to yield physical activities in daily life.

Aging-related attenuation of skeletal muscle mass had been addressed to a smaller muscle fiber size rather than loss of fiber number and characterized of type II myofiber phenotype dominant [13, 40]. In addition, sarcopenic muscles remain in a state of failing compensatory effort in an attempt to stave off muscular degeneration and atrophy [41]. Given the facts that myofiber hypertrophy activated by satellite cells is largely dependent on both net muscle protein synthesis and satellite cell recruitment through serious cellular processing mechanism [42, 43], and that both age-associated sarcopenia and obesity are associated with an over expression of myostatin which functions as a protein inhibitor negatively regulating the skeletal muscle growth and homeostasis with inhibiting the myoblasts proliferation and differentiation [44–46], it is important to identify whether resistance exercises exert any effect on the myofiber type-specific muscle mass loss in obese aged people. In such scenarios, previous trials claimed that age-related Type II myofiber phenotype atrophy would be improved following resistance exercise training by means of satellite cell proliferation and an increase in the rate of muscle contractile and mitochondrial protein synthesis, which further contributed to myofiber hypertrophy [40, 42, 47–51].

Progressive resistance exercise training (RET) has been used as an effective way of improving muscle function and increasing muscle mass by stimulating muscle protein synthesis in elder people [31, 49, 52, 53]. Liao et al. further indicate that elastic RET exerts benefits on lean mass and physical mobility in older women with sarcopenic obesity [54]. With respective to multidisciplinary interventions for prevention of sarcopenia in elder populations, an additional protein supplements (PS) has also been believed to augment the effects of resistance training on muscle mass gain in older adults [55, 56]. For obese elderly individuals with energy restricted diet, PS has its effect on reduction of losing muscle mass during caloric restriction-induced weight loss [57]. However, the effects of PS plus RET on muscle mass and strength gains for obese elder people remain controversy. While several studies identified the effects of PS on muscle mass accretion and strength gain during resistance training in sarcopenic or obese elderly individuals [58], some concluded that PS provides no additional benefit in resistance-trained obese elder individuals [59, 60]. Furthermore, few systemic review studies have summarized these results in obese elder individuals. Whether PS during RET exerts any benefit on augmentation of muscular and functional performance in obese elder people remains unclear.

Liao et al. conducted a systemic review and meta-analysis study to investigate effects of PS plus RET for obese elder people [61]. Main results of Liao's study showed an overall effect on lean body mass (LBM) and fat mass with significant standardized mean differences (SMDs) of 0.58 (95% CI = 0.32, 0.84, $P < 0.0001$) and − 0.61 (95% CI = −0.93, −0.29; $P = 0.0002$) favoring PS plus RET, respectively; similar results were observed in leg strength (SMD = 0.69, 95% CI = 0.39, 0.98; $P < 0.00001$) and short physical performance battery test (SMD = 0.44, 95% CI = 0.11, 0.78, $P = 0.009$). The results indicate that PS during RET intervention may potentially positively contribute to changes in the body composition of overweight and obese older people. However, based on the lower body mass index (BMI) subgroup (mean BMI < 30 kg/m^2) exhibited greater changes in muscle volume and handgrip strength whereas the subgroup with mean BMI ≥ 30 kg/m^2 did not after PS, obese older individuals may be resistant to PS to some degree [61].

2.2 Associations of muscle mass changes with intervention effects on muscle strength and physical capability after protein supplement plus exercise training

Multidisciplinary approaches are recommended for elderly individuals who have high sarcopenia or frailty risks, including nutrient intervention alone, exercise training alone, or combination of both [62–66], and among which protein supplement combined with exercise training (PS + ET) has been widely employed to augment lean mass gain, strength gain, and physical function enhancement in elderly individuals, irrespective of PS types and exercise protocols [65, 67–69]. However, whether intervention-induced changes in muscle mass contribute to strength gain and physical mobility improvement after PS + ET remains unclear. Several previous meta-analysis studies have reported that an increase in lean mass is accompanied by significant increases in strength gain [61, 68, 70–72] as well as physical mobility [68, 72] following PS + ET; however, such simultaneous increases in lean mass with strength [67, 73] (or physical function [61, 71]) were not observed by other researchers. Low muscle mass strongly predicts strength loss and mobility limitations in older adults [17, 74]; in addition, sarcopenia has been addressed to suppressed muscle protein turnover and homeostasis [75, 76]; therefore, identification of relationship between the muscle mass changes and physical improvements in response to PS + ET can facilitate clinical practitioners to efficiently make optimal decisions and set appropriate intervention strategies for elderly patients who are diagnosed as sarcopenia or frailty.

Liao et al. conducted a systemic review and meta-regression study to determine the associations of lean mass changes with treatment effects on strength and physical mobility after PS + ET [77]. Main results of Liao's study showed an overall effect on LBM and appendicular lean mass (ALM) with significant SMDs of 0.66 (95%CI: 0.41–0.91, $P < 0.00001$) and 0.40 (95%CI: 0.15–0.66, $P = 0.002$) favoring PS + ET, respectively; similar results were observed in leg strength (SMD = 0.65, 95% CI:

0.39–0.90; $P < 0.00001$) and walking capability (SMD = 0.33, 95% CI: 0.14–0.52; $P = 0.0006$). Meta-regression analysis results of Liao's study showed that significant associations were observed between changes in ALM ($\beta = 0.08$, $P = 0.003$) and SMDs of leg strength; the results further indicated that elderly individuals who achieved an increase in ALM of >2.5% in response to PS + ET may have obtained a positive effect size of leg strength. In addition, changes in ALM were significantly associated with effect sizes of walking capability ($\beta = 0.17$, $P = 0.04$). According to the Liao's results, intervention-induced muscle mass gains have contributions in strength gain and function recovery after PS + ET, particularly the elderly who have sarcopenia and frailty risks.

3. Management of muscle deficits for mild to moderate severity of osteoarthritis

Since OA has been recognized as a serious musculoskeletal disease [78], managements of OA comprise multidisciplinary interventions including pain medications and nonpharmacological treatments for those patients who exhibit mild to moderate symptoms. However, surgical treatments such as total joint arthroplasty that could help to relief pain and improve joint function (e.g., range of motion and strength) [79] are commonly recommended at the end stage of OA.

Evidences regarding the effects of ET alone or PS plus ET on muscle mass, strength, and physical mobility have been well established in elderly populations with sarcopenia (**Figure 1**). However, whether ET alone or PS plus ET exert any benefit on muscle mass and function outcomes remains unclear. Based on that low muscle mass is closely associated with OA and elder individuals with OA have high sarcopenia risk [10, 28], it is urgent to generate effective strategy to manage this condition for the rapidly growing OA population. In addition, it is necessary

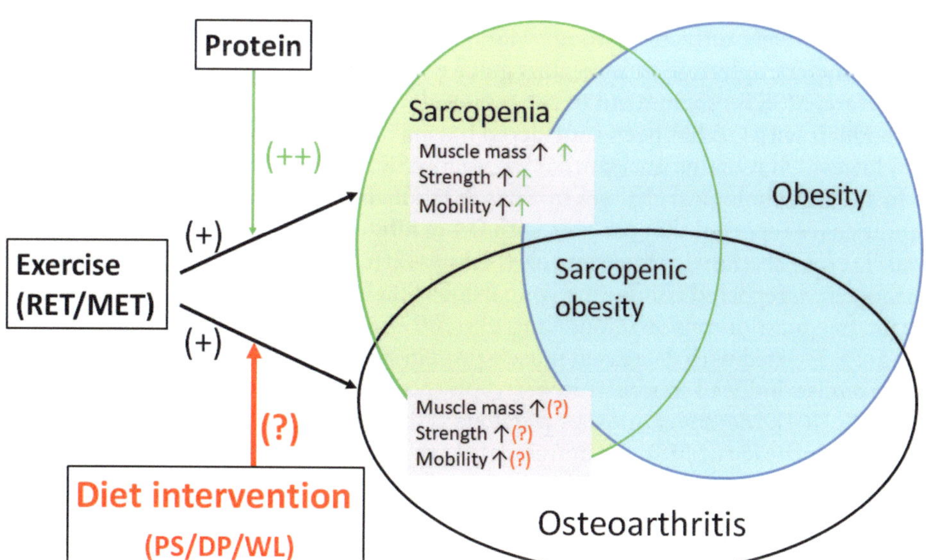

Figure 1.
Summary of evidences regarding effects of exercise and diet interventions on sarcopenia, sarcopenic obesity, and osteoarthritis. Black, green, and red arrow lines indicate exercise alone, protein supplement plus exercise, and diet interventions plus exercise, respectively. (+): significant intervention effect; (++): significantly additional effect; (?) unclear additional effect. RET, resistance exercise training; MET, multicomponent exercise training; PS, protein supplement; DP, dietary protein; WL, weight loss.

to identify evidence of intervention effects on muscle mass and strength gains for elder people with OA.

3.1 Exercise training

Among the interventions of OA, exercise therapy is recommended as one of the first-line treatments [80]. Exercise exerts benefits on pain reduction, muscle strength, and physical function in elder individuals with OA, regardless of exercise types [81]. Especially, the muscle strength-based exercise training (MSE) has been encouraged to minimize degenerative muscular function associated with aging [82, 83], because of that elder individuals experience well muscular adaptations in terms of muscle morphological and architectural changes responding to MSE [84]. Therefore, MSE has been recommended for elder people with OA to augment muscle volume and enhance muscle hypertrophy [80].

Previous results have shown that MSE exerts benefits on muscle mass gain in elderly people. Churchward-Venne et al. indicated that older individuals achieved significantly temporal changes in whole body lean mass at 12-week and 24-week follow up by 0.9 ± 0.1 kg ($P < 0.001$) and 1.1 ± 0.2 kg ($P < 0.001$), respectively, responding to prolonged resistance-type MSE with an intensity of 60–80% 1RM and an intervention duration of 24 weeks [85]. In a meta-analysis, Peterson et al. indicated that resistance exercise exerts significant effects on increasing LBM with a pooled mean difference of 1.1 kg (95% CI: 0.9–1.2 kg) compared to the controls in older people [53].

The MSE has been served as the most promising intervention for sarcopenic elderly [62, 86] as well as those with OA [87–90] to increase strength and improve mobility. Due to that MSE enables older adults to yield increased muscle anabolic resistance occurring with advancing age [91, 92], resistance-type exercise training (RET) as well as multicomponent exercise training (MET) have been considered beneficial for preserving lean muscle mass in older populations, even in those with sarcopenia [53, 93]. In addition, muscle protein synthesis and myofiber proliferation can be effectively activated through MSE [94], which further contribute to skeletal muscle hypertrophy and muscle mass gains even in elder population [42, 43]. Therefore, MSE is recommend to be employed for management of OA since elder individuals with OA has been considered having low muscle mass [10].

However, it remains unclear that whether MSE has any effect on muscle mass gain and morphological changes in older individuals with lower extremities of OA. Studies have reported that patients with OA exhibited increased changes in the muscle cross-sectional area or muscle thickness after MSE [95–97], whereas other authors have reported conflicting conclusions that MSE exerted no beneficial effects on fat-free mass or muscle remodeling [98–100]. In addition, both sarcopenia and OA are associated with decreased muscle protein synthesis and homeostasis [75, 76], and exercise-induced muscular hypertrophy contributes to the increase of muscle strength [101]. Moreover, most of previous systematic reviews investigating the treatment efficacy of MSE for individuals with OA have focused on muscular strength and physical outcomes rather than the muscle mass or volume measures [87–90]. Therefore, identifying the effects of MSE on increasing muscle mass and volume helps clinical practitioners to develop appropriate treatment strategies for older people with OA.

Liao et al. conducted a systemic review and meta-analysis study to investigate effects of MSE for elder people with lower extremity OA [77]. Main results of systemic review and meta-analyses showed MSE has effects on changes in muscle mass gain (SMD = 0.49, 95% CI: 0.28, 0.71; $P < 0.00001$), muscle thickness (SMD = 0.82, 95% CI: 0.20, 1.43; $P = 0.009$), and muscle cross-sectional area (SMD = 0.80, 95%

CI: 0.25, 1.35; $P = 0.004$) compared with nonexercise controls. Liao's study demonstrated that MSE exerts effects on lean mass gain as well as muscle morphological changes in older adults with knee or hip OA. In addition, the subgroup analysis results suggested that older men experienced greater MSE effects on muscle thickness than did women peers and those who received MSE after arthroplasty may achieve greater changes in muscle volume compared to those who received preoperative an MSE intervention or those who did not undergo arthroplasty. According to the results in Liao's meta-analysis, MSE may aid in offsetting muscle attenuation or prevent sarcopenia in older individuals with knee or hip OA, particularly in older men and in those undergoing knee or hip arthroplasty.

3.2 Protein supplement

Diet intervention such as dietary protein or protein supplementation (PS) has been incorporated to multidisciplinary managements for OA [102], since elder patients with OA have potential risks of age-related sarcopenia. In addition, alternative and complementary therapeutic approaches, such as the use of a wide array of nutritional and physical manipulations, are becoming popular for relieving symptoms of OA. Several previous studies had investigated clinical efficacy of protein supplementation (PS) for elder individuals with knee OA [103–106]. Colker et al. employed a 6-week milk PS for elder individuals with OA and the results showed that PS achieved significant improved changes of daily activity and the Western Ontario and McMaster Universities Osteoarthritis Index (WOMAC) per week compared with the placebo group ($P < 0.001$) [104]; Zenk et al. conducted a similar study for older adults with OA and demonstrated that compared with the placebo supplement, a 6-week milk PS obtained significant effects on WOMAC and reduction of medication use as well as the glucosamine-supplement group did [106]. Arjmandi et al. further indicated that a 3-month soy-protein supplement achieved greater changes in pain, physical difficulty, and medical requirement than milk PS did, particularly for elder men with OA [103]. Regarding other types of PS, Miller et al. used an alternative PS of leucine enriched herbal and indicated that WOMAC and pain score were significantly reduced in PS group by 15% ($P < 0.05$) and 21.8% ($P < 0.002$), respectively, compared to the placebo group (reduced 25.4% in WOMAC and 21.8% in pain) [105].

3.3 Protein supplement combined with exercise training

Nutritional intervention, especially the protein supplementation (PS), can influence outcomes for elder individuals undergoing exercise interventions such as resistance-based exercise training (RET) or multicomponent exercise training (MET). Several systematic review studies had identified benefits of PS plus exercise training for elder population. For healthy elder individuals, Morton et al. reported that prolonged PS plus RET has effects on fat free mass, mid-thigh cross-sectional area, and one-repetition maximum strength by significant pooled mean differences of 0.30 kg (95%CI: 0.09–0.52 kg; $P = 0.007$), 7.2 mm^2 (95%CI: 0.20–14.30 mm^2; $P = 0.04$), and 2.49 kg (95%CI: 0.64–4.33 kg; $P = 0.01$), respectively [67]. For overweight or obese elder individuals, Liao et al. indicated that PS plus RET exerts significant effects on LBM and muscle volume with the corresponding effect sizes being 0.58 (95% CI: 0.32–0.84; $P < 0.0001$) and 1.23 (95% CI: 0.50–1.96; $P = 0.001$), respectively, irrespective of the intervention period [61]. For frail elderly, Liao et al. demonstrated that PS plus either RET or MET exerts significant effects on LBM and leg strength with the corresponding effect sizes being 0.52 (95% CI: 0.33–0.71; $P < 0.00001$) and 0.37 (95% CI: 0.23–0.51; $P < 0.00001$), respectively [68]. According to the previous established evidence regarding efficacy of PS plus exercise training, additional PS employed during exercise training may exert benefits for elder population with OA. However, most of the previous systematic review and meta-analysis studies investigated effects of PS plus exercise training for sarcopenic or frail elderly people, few studies focusing on OA population who are potentially with a high risk of sarcopenia. Further studies are necessary to investigate treatment effects of PS plus exercise on elderly population with OA.

3.4 Weight loss plus exercise for sarcopenic obesity in osteoarthritis

Given that obesity has become a burden in OA population [25], weight loss (WL) should be considered as an option while setting the treatment goals and planning rehabilitation strategies for elder people with OA. Previous studies had shown that maintaining or lowering BMI to the normal range (usually within 20.0–24.9, regardless of ethic) may reduce risks or improve symptoms of OA [107, 108]. Felson et al. indicated that a decrease of over 50% in odds of developing OA (odds ratio = 0.46; $P = 0.02$) occurred in older women along with a 2-unit decrease in BMI or a 5.1-kg reduction in weight over a 10-year period, especially for those who had a baseline BMI > 25 kg/m^2 (odds ratio = 0.41; $P = 0.02$) [108]. Coggon et al. concluded similar results that proportion of knee OA patients can be reduced from 10.9 to 57.1% while overweight and obese populations reduced their weight by 2–5 kg or until reaching the normal-range BMI [107]. Weight loss is also efficacious in relieving symptoms of knee OA, most importantly alleviating the pain. Riddle et al. observed a significant dose-response relationship ($P < 0.003$) exists between percentage changes in body weight and the corresponding changes in WOMAC pain, as well as WOMAC physical function; Riddle further indicated that weight changes (gain or loss) of ≥10% potentially leads to clinical important changes in pain and function for older individuals with OA [109]. Messier et al. also identified a dose response to WL for pain ($P = 0.01$), 6-minute walk distance ($P < 0.0001$), and function ($P = 0.0006$) [110]. Accordingly, WL should be incorporated to the management for elder individuals with OA, especially those who are overweight or obese.

An WL intervention may exert negative impacts on lean mass since obesity often masks the age-associated loss of muscle mass. Recently, WL in combination with exercise has been recommended as the optimal approach to managing obese patients with OA. Several previous trials had targeted weight management for obese older adults with OA including the Intensive Diet and Exercise for Arthritis Trial [111], the Arthritis, Diet and Activity Promotion Trial [112], and the Physical Activity, Inflammation, and Body Composition Trial [113]. These registered clinical trials employed weight-loss protocols which targeted 5–10% reduction of body weight over 6–18 months and incorporated partial meal replacements, nutrition class, and behavior therapy for diet habit changes and lifestyle modifications. Results from such previous trials showed that exercise training in combination with a weight-loss program in obese adults with knee OA achieved significantly greater changes in pain and function compared to the control groups. In addition, several systemic reviews regarding WL with or without exercise for elder OA populations also provide evidences for treatment efficacy on pain relief and function recovery [114–117]. However, the effects of WL plus exercise on lean mass remain inconsistency among the results of previous trials and few systemic review and meta-analysis studies focused on the treatment efficacy on muscle mass outcome in obese elder individuals with OA who received WL plus exercise. Future studies should be warranted to investigate effects of WL plus exercise on muscle mass in order to prevent sarcopenia in such elder population with OA.

Liao et al. conducted a systemic review and meta-analysis study to investigate effects of diet intervention plus ET for elder people with mild to moderate OA [118]. Among the included trials in Liao's study, all of the included trials which reported muscle mass outcomes conducted a WL plus ET intervention for obese elder patients with knee OA [118] and the results showed that during an overall follow-up duration, the WL plus ET group achieved significant effects on muscle mass gains (SMD = 0.61; 95%CI: 0.30–0.91, P = 0.0001) compared to the control groups, regardless of methodological design. The results indicated that WL plus ET exhibited significant effects on muscle mass for obese older individuals with OA.

4. Management of muscle dysfunction after total joint replacement for patients with end-stage osteoarthritis

4.1 Postoperative rehabilitation for muscle recovery after total joint replacement

Total joint replacement has been recommended for patients with end-stage of OA who experience poor response to pharmacological medication or conventional therapy [119–121]. Total knee replacement (TKR) as well as total hip replacement (THR) has profound benefits for pain relief, which is the main determinant of functional recovery following surgery.

Enhanced recovery programs after a TKR or THR surgery, which require a multidisciplinary team of dedicated professionals, have been well-established [122]. Among the perioperative interventions producing better surgery outcome, rehabilitation plays an important role in physical reconditioning and functional recovery [123]. As mentioned in the Section 2.1, muscle strengthening exercise (MSE) exerts benefits on muscle mass and strength gains in elder people with OA, and an MSE has been effectively employed following TKR or THR surgery as well to improve postoperative muscle and joint function [124]. However, it remains unclear that whether MSE exerts any effect on muscle mass after total joint replacement. It is important to identify the effects of MSE on muscle mass outcome following total joint replacement since patient who were undergoing TKR or THR may experience acute sarcopenia immediately after surgery [125, 126]. Due to that sarcopenia may have impacts on function outcome after TKR or THR, further studies should be conducted to warrant effective interventions for preserve muscle mass for elderly population with OA who recently underwent total joint replacement.

Liao et al. conducted a randomized control trial to investigate effects of post-TKR MSE for elder women with OA [127]. Liao's study demonstrated that an intervention of 12-week elastic RET following TKR surgery exerted benefits for muscle mass gain and physical recovery among elderly women with KOA. The results of this study suggest that elastic RET should be incorporated to post-TKR rehabilitation for patients with KOA to achieve well postoperative outcomes, especially muscle mass gains and physical mobility improvements. Liao further stated that the elastic RET is relatively safe and easily performed at home. The elastic RET protocol used in Liao's study will help clinical practitioners and physiotherapists and to establish prompt treatment strategies for elderly people with KOA, especially those who have undergone a recent TKR and are considered to have high sarcopenia risk. The findings of this study indicated post-TKR elastic RET exerted benefits on muscle mass and function and can potentially assist clinician decision-making concerning the optimal treatment strategy for elderly women who are undergoing a primary TKR.

4.2 Protein supplement plus exercise training after surgery

The previous observational study has indicated that low protein intake occurring in patients with OA may place themselves at high risks of sarcopenia [128]. Therefore, perioperative interventions including protein supplement may prevent elder patients from suffering acute sarcopenia and poor surgical outcome at early stage after total joint replacement (i.e., TKR or THR) [129–131]. Alito et al. employed 5-day protein-contained (23%) supplements (PS) before surgery for patients who were undergoing THR and the results demonstrated that comparing with the non-supplement control group, the PS group experienced significantly a lower level of C-reactive protein (mean 80.6 vs. 66.5 mg/L, $P < 0.01$) and a shorter length of hospital stay (median 6 vs. 3 days, $P < 0.01$) after THR [129]. Yang et al. used high-dose PS on the day before and after THR surgery and the results showed that, comparing to the standard-care group, the PS group had less proportion of patients who required an intravenous albumin (45.1% vs. 26.8%, $P = 0.023$) and experienced a shorter length of hospital stay (mean 5.1 vs. 3.9 days, $P < 0.001$) [130]. Bai et al. used an oral ingestion of hydrolyzed PS for 5 postoperative days after TKR and the results indicated that PS enhanced postoperative nutrition status in terms of greater changes in blood prealbumin ($P < 0.03$) compared to the regular-nutrition group [131]. The previous results had indicated that diet interventions, especially the PS, before or after total joint replacement can enhance postoperative nutrient status and shorten length of acute inpatient stay which further prevent elder patients from experiencing acute sarcopenia.

On the basis that either perioperative diet interventions or early rehabilitation programs exerts benefits on surgical outcome, combination of both may provide additional effects on function recovery after TKR or THR. The evidences regarding effects of PS plus exercise for healthy, sarcopenic, and frail elder populations have been well established by previous systemic review and meta-analysis studies [61, 68, 132]. However, the elder population with OA as well as those who underwent total joint replacement are less targeted by previous systemic reviews investigating efficacy of PS plus exercise. Future studies are necessary to be warranted in order to identify whether PS plus exercise following TKR or THR exerts any effect on postoperative function outcomes.

Liao et al. conducted a systemic review and meta-analysis study to investigate effects of diet intervention plus ET for elder people with OA [118]. Among the included trials in Liao's study, all of the included trials which reported muscle mass outcomes conducted a PS plus ET intervention for older patients who recently received a TKR or THR [118] and the results showed that during an overall follow-up duration, the PS plus ET group achieved significant effects on muscle mass gains (SMD = 0.81; 95%CI: 0.45–1.17, $P < 0.0001$) compared to the ET control groups, regardless of PS type. The results indicated that PS plus ET exhibited significant effects on muscle mass for older individuals with OA, especially for those who recently received a total joint arthroplasty.

5. Conclusions

This review provides evidence that DI incorporated with ET is effective for promoting gains in muscle mass and strength and enhancing performance in physical mobility for the elder adults with lower-extremity OA, compared to placebo, DI-alone or ET-alone controls. In addition, muscle mass gains have effects on strength gain and global function recovery. Furthermore, the results of this study showed that PS plus ET appears to be the optimal treatment strategy for those who were undergoing total joint replacement whereas WL plus ET is most preferred for those who experienced mild to moderate severity of OA disease. Therefore, we concluded that DI additional to ET may have extra effects to prevent or offset muscle loss and function decline for elder individuals with OA who have high sarcopenia risks.

6. Implications for clinical practice

This review adds current evidences of interdisciplinary approach practices which comprise effective nutrient and exercise intervention strategies for KOA populations who have potential risks of sarcopenic obesity. This review also provides references for clinical practitioners to develop efficient and effective interventions for such population to prevent sarcopenic obesity.

Acknowledgements

This study was funded by grants from the Taipei Medical University-Shuang Ho Hospital, Ministry of Health and Welfare, Taiwan (grant no. 109TMU-SHH-13) and Taipei Medical University (grant no. IIT-1072-3).

Conflict of interest

The authors declare that they have no conflict of interest to the publication of this review.

Author details

Tsan-Hon Liou[1]*, Chun-De Liao[2] and Shih-Wei Huang[1]

1 Department of Physical Medicine and Rehabilitation, School of Medicine, College of Medicine, Taipei Medical University, Taipei, Taiwan

2 Department of Physical Medicine and Rehabilitation, Shuang Ho Hospital, Taipei Medical University, Taipei, Taiwan

*Address all correspondence to: peter_liou@s.tmu.edu.tw

References

[1] United Nations, D.o.E.a.S.A., Population Division. World Population Prospects 2019: Ten Key Findings. 2019. 25 October 2019. Available from: https://population.un.org/wpp/Publications/Files/WPP2019_10KeyFindings.pdf

[2] Guzman-Castillo M et al. Forecasted trends in disability and life expectancy in England and Wales up to 2025: A modelling study. The Lancet Public Health. 2017;**2**(7):e307-e313

[3] Palazzo C et al. Respective contribution of chronic conditions to disability in France: Results from the national disability-health survey. PLoS One. 2012;**7**(9):e44994

[4] Prince MJ et al. The burden of disease in older people and implications for health policy and practice. The Lancet. 2015;**385**(9967):549-562

[5] Sebbag E et al. The world-wide burden of musculoskeletal diseases: A systematic analysis of the World Health Organization burden of diseases database. Annals of the Rheumatic Diseases. 2019;**78**(6):844-848

[6] Palazzo C et al. The burden of musculoskeletal conditions. PLoS One. 2014;**9**(3):e90633

[7] Cruz-Jentoft AJ et al. Sarcopenia: Revised European consensus on definition and diagnosis. Age and Ageing. 2019;**48**(1):16-31

[8] Rolland Y et al. Difficulties with physical function associated with obesity, sarcopenia, and sarcopenic-obesity in community-dwelling elderly women: The EPIDOS (EPIDemiologie de l'OSteoporose) study. The American Journal of Clinical Nutrition. 2009;**89**(6):1895-1900

[9] Kim SR et al. Associations between fat mass, lean mass, and knee osteoarthritis: The fifth Korean National Health and nutrition examination survey (KNHANES V). Calcified Tissue International. 2016;**99**(6):598-607

[10] Kim HT et al. An analysis of age-related loss of skeletal muscle mass and its significance on osteoarthritis in a Korean population. The Korean Journal of Internal Medicine. 2016;**31**(3):585-593

[11] Tieland M, Trouwborst I, Clark BC. Skeletal muscle performance and ageing. Journal of Cachexia, Sarcopenia and Muscle. 2018;**9**(1):3-19

[12] Kwan P. Sarcopenia, a neurogenic syndrome? Journal of Aging Research. 2013;**2013**:791679

[13] Nilwik R et al. The decline in skeletal muscle mass with aging is mainly attributed to a reduction in type II muscle fiber size. Experimental Gerontology. 2013;**48**(5):492-498

[14] Mitchell WK et al. Sarcopenia, dynapenia, and the impact of advancing age on human skeletal muscle size and strength; a quantitative review. Frontiers in Physiology. 2012;**3**:260

[15] Wilkinson DJ, Piasecki M, Atherton PJ. The age-related loss of skeletal muscle mass and function: Measurement and physiology of muscle fibre atrophy and muscle fibre loss in humans. Ageing Research Reviews. 2018;**47**:123-132

[16] Reid KF et al. Lower extremity muscle mass predicts functional performance in mobility-limited elders. The Journal of Nutrition, Health & Aging. 2008;**12**(7):493-498

[17] Liu LK et al. Age-related skeletal muscle mass loss and physical performance in Taiwan: Implications to diagnostic strategy of sarcopenia

in Asia. Geriatrics & Gerontology International. 2013;**13**(4):964-971

[18] Malmstrom TK et al. Low appendicular skeletal muscle mass (ASM) with limited mobility and poor health outcomes in middle-aged African Americans. Journal of Cachexia, Sarcopenia and Muscle. 2013;**4**(3):179-186

[19] Toda Y et al. A decline in lower extremity lean body mass per body weight is characteristic of women with early phase osteoarthritis of the knee. The Journal of Rheumatology. 2000;**27**(10):2449-2454

[20] Lee SY et al. Low skeletal muscle mass in the lower limbs is independently associated to knee osteoarthritis. PLoS One. 2016;**11**(11):e0166385

[21] Jeon H et al. Low skeletal muscle mass and radiographic osteoarthritis in knee, hip, and lumbar spine: A cross-sectional study. Aging Clinical and Experimental Research. 2019;**31**(11):1557-1562

[22] Shorter E et al. Skeletal muscle wasting and its relationship with osteoarthritis: A mini-review of mechanisms and current interventions. Current Rheumatology Reports. 2019;**21**(8):40

[23] Grimaldi A et al. The association between degenerative hip joint pathology and size of the gluteus medius, gluteus minimus and piriformis muscles. Manual Therapy. 2009;**14**(6):605-610

[24] Zacharias A et al. Atrophy of hip abductor muscles is related to clinical severity in a hip osteoarthritis population. Clinical Anatomy. 2018;**31**(4):507-513

[25] Lechleitner M. The elderly as a target for obesity treatment. Expert Review of Endocrinology and Metabolism. 2015;**10**(4):375-380

[26] Batsis JA et al. Impact of obesity on disability, function, and physical activity: Data from the osteoarthritis initiative. Scandinavian Journal of Rheumatology. 2015;**44**(6):495-502

[27] Ackerman IN, Osborne RH. Obesity and increased burden of hip and knee joint disease in Australia: Results from a national survey. BMC Musculoskeletal Disorders. 2012;**13**:254

[28] Kemmler W et al. Prevalence of sarcopenia in Germany and the corresponding effect of osteoarthritis in females 70 years and older living in the community: Results of the FORMoSA study. Clinical Interventions in Aging. 2015;**10**:1565-1573

[29] Jin C et al. The clinical research of rehabilitation method based on virtual reality technology for early functional exercise after total knee arthroplasty. Chinese Journal of Control of Endemic Diseases. 2017;**32**(7):779-780

[30] Misra D et al. Risk of knee osteoarthritis with obesity, sarcopenic obesity, and sarcopenia. Arthritis & Rhematology. 2019;**71**(2):232-237

[31] Vincent HK, Raiser SN, Vincent KR. The aging musculoskeletal system and obesity-related considerations with exercise. Ageing Research Reviews. 2012;**11**(3):361-373

[32] Choi KM. Sarcopenia and sarcopenic obesity. Endocrinology and Metabolism. 2013;**28**(2):86-89

[33] Molino S et al. Sarcopenic obesity: An appraisal of the current status of knowledge and management in elderly people. The Journal of Nutrition, Health & Aging. 2016;**20**(7):780-788

[34] Deutz NE et al. Protein intake and exercise for optimal muscle function with aging: Recommendations from the ESPEN expert group. Clinical Nutrition. 2014;**33**(6):929-936

[35] von Haehling S, Morley JE, Anker SD. From muscle wasting to sarcopenia and myopenia: Update 2012. Journal of Cachexia, Sarcopenia and Muscle. 2012;**3**(4):213-217

[36] Visser M et al. Leg muscle mass and composition in relation to lower extremity performance in men and women aged 70 to 79: The health, aging and body composition study. Journal of the American Geriatrics Society. 2002;**50**(5):897-904

[37] Zoico E et al. Physical disability and muscular strength in relation to obesity and different body composition indexes in a sample of healthy elderly women. International Journal of Obesity and Related Metabolic Disorders. 2004;**28**(2):234-241

[38] Vincent HK, Vincent KR, Lamb KM. Obesity and mobility disability in the older adult. Obesity Reviews. 2010;**11**(8):568-579

[39] Lee S, Kim TN, Kim SH. Sarcopenic obesity is more closely associated with knee osteoarthritis than is nonsarcopenic obesity: A cross-sectional study. Arthritis and Rheumatism. 2012;**64**(12):3947-3954

[40] Verdijk LB et al. Skeletal muscle hypertrophy following resistance training is accompanied by a fiber type-specific increase in satellite cell content in elderly men. The Journals of Gerontology. Series A, Biological Sciences and Medical Sciences. 2009;**64**(3):332-339

[41] Calvani R et al. Mitochondrial pathways in sarcopenia of aging and disuse muscle atrophy. Biological Chemistry. 2013;**394**(3):393-414

[42] Damas F et al. A review of resistance training-induced changes in skeletal muscle protein synthesis and their contribution to hypertrophy. Sports Medicine. 2015;**45**(6):801-807

[43] Zammit PS, Partridge TA, Yablonka-Reuveni Z. The skeletal muscle satellite cell: The stem cell that came in from the cold. The Journal of Histochemistry and Cytochemistry. 2006;**54**(11):1177-1191

[44] Elliott B et al. The central role of myostatin in skeletal muscle and whole body homeostasis. Acta Physiologica (Oxford, England). 2012;**205**(3):324-440

[45] Allen DL, Hittel DS, McPherron AC. Expression and function of myostatin in obesity, diabetes, and exercise adaptation. Medicine and Science in Sports and Exercise. 2011;**43**(10):1828-1835

[46] Yarasheski KE et al. Serum myostatin-immunoreactive protein is increased in 60-92 year old women and men with muscle wasting. The Journal of Nutrition, Health & Aging. 2002;**6**(5):343-348

[47] Farup J, Sorensen H, Kjolhede T. Similar changes in muscle fiber phenotype with differentiated consequences for rate of force development: Endurance versus resistance training. Human Movement Science. 2014;**34**:109-119

[48] Kosek DJ et al. Efficacy of 3 days/wk resistance training on myofiber hypertrophy and myogenic mechanisms in young vs. older adults. Journal of Applied Physiology. 1985;**101**(2):531-544

[49] Yarasheski KE. Exercise, aging, and muscle protein metabolism. The Journals of Gerontology. Series A, Biological Sciences and Medical Sciences. 2003;**58**(10):M918-M922

[50] Melov S et al. Resistance exercise reverses aging in human skeletal muscle. PLoS One. 2007;**2**(5):e465

[51] Johnston AP, De Lisio M, Parise G. Resistance training, sarcopenia, and the mitochondrial theory of aging. Applied Physiology, Nutrition, and Metabolism. 2008;**33**(1):191-199

[52] Liu CJ, Latham NK. Progressive resistance strength training for improving physical function in older adults. Cochrane Database of Systematic Reviews. 2009;**3**:CD002759

[53] Peterson MD, Sen A, Gordon PM. Influence of resistance exercise on lean body mass in aging adults: A meta-analysis. Medicine and Science in Sports and Exercise. 2011;**43**(2):249-258

[54] Liao CD et al. Effects of elastic band exercise on lean mass and physical capacity in older women with sarcopenic obesity: A randomized controlled trial. Scientific Reports. 2018;**8**(1):2317

[55] Cermak NM et al. Protein supplementation augments the adaptive response of skeletal muscle to resistance-type exercise training: A meta-analysis. The American Journal of Clinical Nutrition. 2012;**96**(6):1454-1464

[56] Tieland M et al. Protein supplementation increases muscle mass gain during prolonged resistance-type exercise training in frail elderly people: A randomized, double-blind, placebo-controlled trial. Journal of the American Medical Directors Association. 2012;**13**(8):713-719

[57] Coker RH et al. Whey protein and essential amino acids promote the reduction of adipose tissue and increased muscle protein synthesis during caloric restriction-induced weight loss in elderly, obese individuals. Nutrition Journal. 2012;**11**(1):105-111

[58] Zdzieblik D et al. Collagen peptide supplementation in combination with resistance training improves body composition and increases muscle strength in elderly sarcopenic men: A randomised controlled trial. The British Journal of Nutrition. 2015;**114**(8):1237-1245

[59] Villanueva MG, He J, Schroeder ET. Periodized resistance training with and without supplementation improve body composition and performance in older men. European Journal of Applied Physiology. 2014;**114**(5):891-905

[60] Verreijen AM et al. A high whey protein-, leucine-, and vitamin D-enriched supplement preserves muscle mass during intentional weight loss in obese older adults: A double-blind randomized controlled trial. American Journal of Clinical Nutrition. 2015;**101**(2):279-286

[61] Liao CD et al. Effects of protein supplementation combined with resistance exercise on body composition and physical function in older adults: A systematic review and meta-analysis. The American Journal of Clinical Nutrition. 2017;**106**(4):1078-1091

[62] Trethewey SP et al. Interventions for the management and prevention of sarcopenia in the critically ill: A systematic review. Journal of Critical Care. 2019;**50**:287-295

[63] Jadczak AD et al. Effectiveness of exercise interventions on physical function in community-dwelling frail older people: An umbrella review of systematic reviews. JBI Database of Systematic Reviews and Implementation Reports. 2018;**16**(3):752-775

[64] Tessier AJ, Chevalier S. An update on protein, leucine, omega-3 fatty acids, and vitamin D in the prevention and treatment of sarcopenia and functional decline. Nutrients. 2018;**10**(8):1099

[65] Phillips SM. Nutritional supplements in support of resistance exercise to counter age-related

sarcopenia. Advances in Nutrition. 2015;**6**(4):452-460

[66] Denison HJ et al. Prevention and optimal management of sarcopenia: A review of combined exercise and nutrition interventions to improve muscle outcomes in older people. Clinical Interventions in Aging. 2015;**10**:859-869

[67] Morton RW et al. A systematic review, meta-analysis and meta-regression of the effect of protein supplementation on resistance training-induced gains in muscle mass and strength in healthy adults. British Journal of Sports Medicine. 2018;**52**(6):376-384

[68] Liao CD et al. Effects of protein supplementation combined with exercise intervention on frailty indices, body composition, and physical function in frail older adults. Nutrients. 2018;**10**(12):1916

[69] Hidayat K et al. Effects of milk proteins supplementation in older adults undergoing resistance training: A meta-analysis of randomized control trials. The Journal of Nutrition, Health & Aging. 2018;**22**(2):237-245

[70] Naclerio F, Larumbe-Zabala E. Effects of whey protein alone or as part of a multi-ingredient formulation on strength, fat-free mass, or lean body mass in resistance-trained individuals: A meta-analysis. Sports Medicine. 2016;**46**(1):125-137

[71] Luo D et al. Effect of nutritional supplement combined with exercise intervention on sarcopenia in the elderly: A meta-analysis. International Journal of Nursing Sciences. 2017;**4**(4):389-401

[72] Cheng H et al. Systematic review and meta-analysis of the effect of protein and amino acid supplements in older adults with acute or chronic conditions. The British Journal of Nutrition. 2018;**119**(5):527-542

[73] Finger D et al. Effects of protein supplementation in older adults undergoing resistance training: A systematic review and meta-analysis. Sports Medicine. 2015;**45**(2):245-255

[74] Janssen I, Heymsfield SB, Ross R. Low relative skeletal muscle mass (sarcopenia) in older persons is associated with functional impairment and physical disability. Journal of the American Geriatrics Society. 2002;**50**(5):889-896

[75] Santos ML et al. Muscle strength, muscle balance, physical function and plasma interleukin-6 (IL-6) levels in elderly women with knee osteoarthritis (OA). Archives of Gerontology and Geriatrics. 2011;**52**(3):322-326

[76] Wilson D et al. Frailty and sarcopenia: The potential role of an aged immune system. Ageing Research Reviews. 2017;**36**:1-10

[77] Liao CD et al. Effects of Muscle Strength Training on Muscle Mass Gain and Hypertrophy in Older Adults with Osteoarthritis: A Systematic Review and Meta-Analysis. Hoboken: Arthritis Care & Research; 2019. DOI: 10.1002/acr.24097 [Online ahead of print]

[78] Hawker GA. Osteoarthritis is a serious disease. Clinical and Experimental Rheumatology. 2019;**120**(5):3-6

[79] Price AJ et al. Knee replacement. Lancet. 2018;**392**(10158):1672-1682

[80] Skou ST, Roos EM. Physical therapy for patients with knee and hip osteoarthritis: Supervised, active treatment is current best practice. Clinical and Experimental Rheumatology. 2019;**37**(5):112-117

[81] Juhl C et al. Impact of exercise type and dose on pain and disability

in knee osteoarthritis: A systematic review and meta-regression analysis of randomized controlled trials. Arthritis & Rhematology. 2014;**66**(3):622-636

[82] Peterson MD, Gordon PM. Resistance exercise for the aging adult: Clinical implications and prescription guidelines. The American Journal of Medicine. 2011;**124**(3):194-198

[83] Giallauria F et al. Resistance training and sarcopenia. Monaldi Archives for Chest Disease. 2016;**84**(1-2):738

[84] Narici MV et al. Muscular adaptations to resistance exercise in the elderly. Journal of Musculoskeletal & Neuronal Interactions. 2004;**4**(2):161-164

[85] Churchward-Venne TA et al. There are no nonresponders to resistance-type exercise training in older men and women. Journal of the American Medical Directors Association. 2015;**16**(5):400-411

[86] Vikberg S et al. Effects of resistance training on functional strength and muscle mass in 70-year-old individuals with pre-sarcopenia: A randomized controlled trial. Journal of the American Medical Directors Association. 2019;**20**(1):28-34

[87] Zacharias A et al. Efficacy of rehabilitation programs for improving muscle strength in people with hip or knee osteoarthritis: A systematic review with meta-analysis. Osteoarthritis and Cartilage. 2014;**22**(11):1752-1773

[88] Jansen MJ et al. Strength training alone, exercise therapy alone, and exercise therapy with passive manual mobilisation each reduce pain and disability in people with knee osteoarthritis: A systematic review. Journal of Physiotherapy. 2011;**57**(1):11-20

[89] Bartholdy C et al. The role of muscle strengthening in exercise therapy for knee osteoarthritis: A systematic review and meta-regression analysis of randomized trials. Seminars in Arthritis and Rheumatism. 2017;**47**(1):9-21

[90] Li Y et al. The effects of resistance exercise in patients with knee osteoarthritis: A systematic review and meta-analysis. Clinical Rehabilitation. 2016;**30**(10):947-959

[91] Agergaard J et al. Light-load resistance exercise increases muscle protein synthesis and hypertrophy signaling in elderly men. American Journal of Physiology. Endocrinology and Metabolism. 2017;**312**(4):E326-E338

[92] Rennie MJ. Anabolic resistance: The effects of aging, sexual dimorphism, and immobilization on human muscle protein turnover. Applied Physiology, Nutrition, and Metabolism. 2009;**34**(3):377-381

[93] Vlietstra L, Hendrickx W, Waters DL. Exercise interventions in healthy older adults with sarcopenia: A systematic review and meta-analysis. Australasian Journal on Ageing. 2018;**37**(3):169-183

[94] Marimuthu K, Murton AJ, Greenhaff PL. Mechanisms regulating muscle mass during disuse atrophy and rehabilitation in humans. Journal of Applied Physiology. 2011;**110**(2):555-560

[95] Ferraz RB et al. Benefits of resistance training with blood flow restriction in knee osteoarthritis. Medicine and Science in Sports and Exercise. 2018;**50**(5):897-905

[96] Mahmoud WS, Elnaggar RK, Ahmed AS. Influence of isometric exercise training on quadriceps muscle architecture and strength in obese subjects with knee osteoarthritis. International Journal of Medical Research & Health Sciences. 2017;**6**(3):1-9

[97] Valtonen A et al. Maintenance of aquatic training-induced benefits on mobility and lower-extremity muscles among persons with unilateral knee replacement. Archives of Physical Medicine and Rehabilitation. 2011;**92**(12):1944-1950

[98] Lim JY, Tchai E, Jang SN. Effectiveness of aquatic exercise for obese patients with knee osteoarthritis: A randomized controlled trial. PM & R : The Journal of Injury, Function, and Rehabilitation. 2010;**2**(8):723-731

[99] Aguiar GC et al. Effects of resistance training in individuals with knee osteoarthritis. Journal of Physical Therapy Science. 2016;**29**(3):589-596

[100] Waller B et al. Effects of high intensity resistance aquatic training on body composition and walking speed in women with mild knee osteoarthritis: A 4-month RCT with 12-month follow-up. Osteoarthritis and Cartilage. 2017;**25**(8):1238-1246

[101] Balshaw TG et al. Changes in agonist neural drive, hypertrophy and pre-training strength all contribute to the individual strength gains after resistance training. European Journal of Applied Physiology. 2017;**117**(4):631-640

[102] Finney A et al. Multidisciplinary approaches to managing osteoarthritis in multiple joint sites: A systematic review. BMC Musculoskeletal Disorders. 2016;**17**:266

[103] Arjmandi BH et al. Soy protein may alleviate osteoarthritis symptoms. Phytomedicine. 2004;**11**(7-8):567-575

[104] Colker CM et al. Effects of a milk-based bioactive micronutrient beverage on pain symptoms and activity of adults with osteoarthritis: A double-blind, placebo-controlled clinical evaluation. Nutrition. 2002;**18**(5):388-392

[105] Miller MJS, Butler R. Relief of osteoarthritis with an herbal-amino acid supplement: A randomized double-blind placebo controlled trial. Advances in Bioscience and Biotechnology. 2012;**3**:504

[106] Zenk JL, Helmer TR, Kuskowski MA. The effects of milk protein concentrate on the symptoms of osteoarthritis in adults: An exploratory, randomized, double-blind, placebo-controlled trial. Current Therapeutic Research. 2002;**63**(7):430-442

[107] Coggon D et al. Knee osteoarthritis and obesity. International Journal of Obesity and Related Metabolic Disorders. 2001;**25**(5):622-627

[108] Felson DT et al. Weight loss reduces the risk for symptomatic knee osteoarthritis in women. The Framingham study. Annals of Internal Medicine. 1992;**116**(7):535-539

[109] Riddle DL, Stratford PW. Body weight changes and corresponding changes in pain and function in persons with symptomatic knee osteoarthritis: A cohort study. Arthritis Care & Research (Hoboken). 2013;**65**(1):15-22

[110] Messier SP et al. Intentional weight loss in overweight and obese patients with knee osteoarthritis: Is more better? Arthritis Care & Research (Hoboken). 2018;**70**(11):1569-1575

[111] Messier SP et al. Effects of intensive diet and exercise on knee joint loads, inflammation, and clinical outcomes among overweight and obese adults with knee osteoarthritis: The IDEA randomized clinical trial. JAMA. 2013;**310**(12):1263-1273

[112] Miller GD et al. The arthritis, diet and activity promotion trial (ADAPT): Design, rationale, and baseline results. Controlled Clinical Trials. 2003;**24**(4):462-480

[113] Miller GD et al. Intensive weight loss program improves physical function in older obese adults with knee osteoarthritis. Obesity (Silver Spring). 2006;**14**(7):1219-1230

[114] Alrushud AS et al. Effect of physical activity and dietary restriction interventions on weight loss and the musculoskeletal function of overweight and obese older adults with knee osteoarthritis: A systematic review and mixed method data synthesis. BMJ Open. 2017;**7**(6):e014537

[115] Christensen R et al. Effect of weight reduction in obese patients diagnosed with knee osteoarthritis: A systematic review and meta-analysis. Annals of the Rheumatic Diseases. 2007;**66**(4):433-439

[116] Chu IJH, Lim AYT, Ng CLW. Effects of meaningful weight loss beyond symptomatic relief in adults with knee osteoarthritis and obesity: A systematic review and meta-analysis. Obesity Reviews. 2018;**19**(11):1597-1607

[117] Robson EK et al. Effectiveness of weight loss interventions for reducing pain and disability in people with common musculoskeletal disorders: A systematic review with meta-analysis. The Journal of Orthopaedic and Sports Physical Therapy. 2020;**50**(6):319-333

[118] Liao CD. Effects of Exercise Training Combined with Diet Intervention for Older Adults with Lower Extremity Osteoarthritis [thesis]. Taipei: National Taiwan University; 2020. DOI: 10.6342/NTU202000990

[119] Liddle AD, Pegg EC, Pandit H. Knee replacement for osteoarthritis. Maturitas. 2013;**75**(2):131-136

[120] Statements NCSS. NIH consensus statement on total knee replacement. NIH Consensus and State-of-the-Science Statements. 2003;**20**(1):1-34

[121] Peters CL. Mild to moderate hip OA: Joint preservation or total hip arthroplasty? The Journal of Arthroplasty. 2015;**30**(7):1109-1112

[122] Ibrahim MS et al. An evidence-based review of enhanced recovery interventions in knee replacement surgery. Annals of the Royal College of Surgeons of England. 2013;**95**(6):386-389

[123] Ebert JR, Munsie C, Joss B. Guidelines for the early restoration of active knee flexion following total knee arthroplasty: implications for rehabilitation and early intervention. Archives of Physical Medicine and Rehabilitation. 2014;**95**(6):1135-1140

[124] Pozzi F, Snyder-Mackler L, Zeni J. Physical exercise after knee arthroplasty: A systematic review of controlled trials. European Journal of Physical and Rehabilitation Medicine. 2013;**49**(6):877-892

[125] Petterson SC et al. Time course of quad strength, area, and activation after knee arthroplasty and strength training. Medicine and Science in Sports and Exercise. 2011;**43**(2):225-231

[126] Kouw IWK et al. One week of hospitalization following elective hip surgery induces substantial muscle atrophy in older patients. Journal of the American Medical Directors Association. 2019;**20**(1):35-42

[127] Liao CD et al. Effects of elastic resistance exercise after total knee replacement on muscle mass and physical function in elderly women with osteoarthritis: A randomized controlled trial. American Journal of Physical Medicine & Rehabilitation. 2020;**99**(5):381-389

[128] de Zwart AH et al. Dietary protein intake and upper leg muscle strength in subjects with knee osteoarthritis:

Data from the osteoarthritis initiative. Rheumatology International. 2019;**39**(2):277-284

[129] Alito MA, de Aguilar-Nascimento JE. Multimodal perioperative care plus immunonutrition versus traditional care in total hip arthroplasty: A randomized pilot study. Nutrition Journal. 2016;**15**:34

[130] Yang L et al. A novel perioperative nutritional management model for primary unilateral total hip arthroplasty. Chinese Journal of Orthopaedics. 2019;**27**(11):1005-1009

[131] Bai ZW et al. Nutritional status improvement in patients undergoing total knee arthroplasty by oral hydrolyzed protein. Beijing Medical Journal. 2018;**40**(1):30-33

[132] Liao CD et al. The role of muscle mass gain following protein supplementation plus exercise therapy in older adults with sarcopenia and frailty risks: A systematic review and meta-regression analysis of randomized trials. Nutrients. 2019;**11**(8):1713